The Joy
Of
Good Health

Rudolph Oehm, M.D.

with

R.A. Oehm

HARVEST HOUSE PUBLISHERS
Irvine, California 92714

The Joy Of Good Health

This book is not intended as a substitute for personalized professional health care. For your individual health-care needs, consult
with your personal physician or other professionally qualified
health-care specialist.

THE JOY OF GOOD HEALTH

CONTENTS

1 THE LIFESAVERS

It was 4 A.M., and Howard awoke with a start. Something seemed to be wrong, but Howard couldn't tell what it was. He felt vaguely uneasy, then thought he must have indigestion, with a little gas building up in the pit of his stomach and under his chest.

Howard thought for another moment, then got up slowly and walked to the kitchen. He took a couple of antacid tablets with water, but that didn't seem to help much, so he went back to bed and tried to rest. As he lay there hoping for relaxation and sleep, the pain seemed to expand into a relentless inner pressure under his breastbone. Howard sat up now, hoping for some relief of the pressure; but instead of diminishing, the pressure now seemed to spread across the entire front of his chest.

Just Something I Ate?

Lois was awake now, and as she looked at Howard somewhat quizzically he responded, "Oh, I'm all right. I think it's just something I ate." Lois looked unconvinced. "Leave me alone," he continued; "I'll be going back to sleep in a minute." Even as he spoke these words, Howard could feel an aching numbness in his left arem. Lois could see the beads of sweat on Howard's face, and she started to leave the bed.

"Where are you going?"

"I'm calling the rescue squad."

"You're doing no such thing!"

"Howard, you're sick!"

"I'm not sick! I just have some heartburn and a muscle cramp.

The bedroom lamp was on now, and Lois looked at Howard's ashen face with alarm. "Howard, you're sick! I'm calling the rescue squad." Howard started to speak again, but before he was able to form the words, he fell from his sitting position to Lois's side of the bed. "Howard, are you all right?" There was no answer. Howard twitched momentarily, then lay totally still.

Call and Breathe

Lois was terrified, but she didn't know what to do. Should she try to help him breathe again, or should she call the rescue squad? Quickly she ran to the phone and dialed the 911 emergency operator. Fortunately, the operator came on quickly, and Lois poured out her emergency in a flow of words. The operator asked her to repeat her problem, and this time Lois spoke more slowly.

As Lois raced back to the bedroom she tried desperately to recall the artificial-respiration technique she had once read about in a ladies' magazine. Was she supposed to pound his chest, or was she supposed to breathe into his mouth? Or was there some other important procedure?

Lois tried to do the simplest thing first. Putting her lips next to Howard's and breathing into his mouth as well as she could, she tried her best, but there seemed to be no response. She was afraid to pound his chest, so she just kept on breathing. Yet Howard's body seemed for all the world like a lifeless corpse.

The Paramedics

Lois heard the distant wail of the siren now, and she breathed a desperate prayer as she ran to the sidewalk to direct the approaching ambulance driver to her house. Seconds later the ambulance doors flew open, and two men carrying strange-looking equipment followed Lois hurriedly into the bedroom. One man snapped open a wheeled litter next to Howard's side of the bed, and then both men moved him gently but quickly onto the flat surface of the litter. One man raised the back of Howard's neck with his hand and began breathing into his mouth, while the other man pressed and released rhythmically on the middle of Howard's chest with the heels of both hands.

Moments later both men began wheeling Howard to the front of the house and into the back of the am-

9

bulance, all the while maintaining their rhythmic chest massage and periodic mouth-to-mouth breathing. One of the men entered the ambulance with Howard, while the other man ran to the driver's seat and slammed the door shut. The neighbors were awake now, and they offered to drive Lois to the hospital just behind the ambulance, so now both vehicles headed for the nearby hospital. Howard's attendant now handled both the chest massaging and the periodic mouth-to-mouth breathing.

Survival!

In a few minutes the ambulance reached the hospital and stopped at the emergency-room entrance. Radio-alerted staff and a doctor were expecting Howard, and he was wheeled quickly from the ambulance to the emergency room. Only seconds later, having already assessed the gravity of the situation, the physician on duty quickly laid two large, paddle-like electrodes on Howard's chest. After everyone had moved clear of the table on which Howard lay, the physician firmly pressed a button on an elaborate machine. Howard's body was jolted with a surge of electrical current, and almost instantly his heart started beating again.

Another attendant resumed artificial respirations with special breathing apparatus, which had been temporarily discontinued because of the defibrillation process. Within a few minutes Howard was breathing on his own adequately enough so that the special breathing apparatus could once more be removed. (By now Howard had also been given intravenous injections of special medications in solution.)

After a few minutes of observation, the attending physician noted that Howard's condition had stabilized, so he allowed Howard to be wheeled to the special coronary care unit of the hospital. Two nurses wheeled him there on a special litter equipped with intravenous drip equipment and a continuous electronic heart monitor. In the coronary care unit Howard was given a continuous intravenous drip of a medication designed to prevent any recurrence of ventricular fibrillation or even any irritability of the heart. In the meantime, the vital statistics of Howard's cardiovascular system were being monitored continuously on special electronic equipment.

Back to Normal?

Though Howard had been continuously unconscious from the time he suffered his heart attack in bed, after about two hours in the special coronary care unit he slowly regained consciousness. At this point Howard could not yet clearly recall the earlier events of the day, but at least he was alive and conscious. During the next few hours the medical staff at the hospital noted that Howard did not appear to have suffered any permanent brain damage, but it was still too early to determine whether his heart would ever allow him to return to his normal activities of life.

2 THE GOAL OF GOOD HEALTH

As Howard lay in his hospital bed during the next several days, both he and Lois learned from the medical staff that he was progressing nicely, with no significant complications. Everyone was encouraged to learn that the damage to Howard's heart, though significant, did not appear to be so massive as to preclude a near-normal life in the months and years ahead. (The paramedics had arrived at Howard's house within about three minutes from his lapse into unconsciousness. Had that figure been four to six minutes or longer, Howard would probably have suffered irreversible brain damage or would have died despite all the most sophisticated rescue efforts.)*

Since far more people in the United States die from heart disease each year than from any other cause (17 times as many as from automobile accidents, for example), we need to ask ourselves, "Is this terrible scourge of death really necessary? Is there anything we

---

* The prompt response of the ambulance attendants and their knowledge of CPR (cardiopulmonary resuscitation) saved Howard's life. In some locations, fully trained paramedics are able to perform even more advanced resuscitation procedures, start intravenous fluids, give medications, and even administer life-saving electrical defibrillation wherever the patient may be found (even before transport). The life-saving technique of CPR can be learned by almost any adult, and even by teenagers at the junior-high level.

can do to prevent heart disease? If we already have
heart disease, is there anything we can do to overcome
it?''

Why Me, God?

As Howard lay in the hospital for the next several
weeks he asked himself, ''Why should this happen to
me? What have I done to deserve such a fate? Is God
punishing me because I'm less religious than I used to
be? Does God really care about me, or does He just
randomly strike down people with heart attacks and
cancer?''

Howard became self-defensive as he thought about
his past. He had been an exceptionally athletic young
man, even playing championship football in his high
school and college years. It's true that he had been a
little overweight for the past several years, but no
more so than the other men in his office. Yes, he
smoked a little, but seldom more than a pack a day.
His blood pressure was a little high, but not nearly as
high as that of two or three of his friends who seemed
to be in robust health. Howard even exercised: once
a week he played 18 holes of golf with several of his
friends from the office. It's true that he rode in the
golf cart more than he walked, but he sure took plenty of swings during the golf games!

Howard did have his business pressures, but who
doesn't have these? And there were the occasional
arguments with Lois and the kids, but what famiy

doesn't go through these from time to time? All in all, Howard felt that his overall life situation was certainly no worse than that of the average male breadwinner and perhaps even somewhat better. For this reason he simply could not understand why he should be subjected to a heart attack that he did not deserve.

The Not-So-Mysterious Killer

Does Howard's life sound like your own life, or perhaps the life of one of your loved ones? If so, read on and learn how you can conquer the not-so-mysterious killer called heart disease.

Each year in the United States nearly a million men and women die from various forms of heart disease. At one time heart disease was thought to be a very mysterious and arbitrary killer of innocent victims, but the immense amount of medical research done in the last 50 years (and most intensely in the last 20 years) has removed much of the mystery from cardiovascular diseases. Before the twentieth century, heart disease was almost never diagnosed properly (partly because it was poorly understood and partly because it occurred less often than today), but with today's continuing research and technology, heart disease is becoming better understood and better diagnosed every year.

If you are willing to learn the basic facts about heart disease as it is understood today, and if you are willing to put these facts into practice in your own life, then you can reasonably expect to live a life that is free from heart attacks, stroke, and several other disabling forms of heart disease. If you already have one or more forms of heart disease, you could well be able to enjoy significant improvement in your health, in some cases dramatically.

Although this book is not intended as a substitute for personalized medical care by your own physician, it can provide you with motivating information and inspiration to help you live a life that is healthy and wholesome as a total person. In this book we will be concentrating not only on overcoming cardiovascular diseases, which include the number one killer in the United States today—heart attack—and the number three killer—stroke—but we will also have something to say about overcoming the number two killer—cancer. The principles of health that apply to these three killers also apply to a number of other diseases which are common in America and the world today, and we would like to show you that the prevention of these diseases is both possible and enjoyable, and that rehabilitation for these diseases is a realistic goal in most cases. Above all, we would like to lead you toward the attainable goal of joyful health in body, soul, and spirit.

What Are the Reasons?

What causes heart attacks? This question has been debated hotly by medical researchers for a number of years, but the underlying causes for heart attacks and other cardiovascular diseases have been emerging more clearly during the last several years. Dozens of sophisticated research projects on heart disease have been undertaken and completed in various parts of the world, and the evidence seems to point rather strongly toward a composite of so-called "risk factors." What this means is that in most cases the onset of heart disease in a particular person can be identified by at least one and usually several factors in combination. What are these factors that contribute to heart attacks? Here they are in their possible order of importance:

1. Age, sex, and heredity
2. Cigarette smoking
3. Abnormal levels of blood fats
4. High blood pressure
5. Lack of exercise
6. Mental stress and Type A personality
7. Diabetes mellitus or glucose intolerance
8. Obesity
9. Miscellaneous

There are probably still other factors that contribute to heart disease, but the ones listed above have been reasonably well-established, especially the first four. The classic Framingham Heart Study put particular emphasis on age, sex, serum cholesterol elevation, hypertension, cigarette smoking, abnormal glucose tolerance, and electrocardiogram abnormalities. But vital capacity (a measurement of lung function) and body weight were also significant, though to a lesser degree. Worldwide studies have helped to confirm these same factors, and to perhaps emphasize some others also.

Actually, most (and perhaps all) of these factors are somewhat interrelated. For example, if you are significantly overweight, you are likely to have higher-than-normal levels of blood cholesterol, blood pressure, and blood sugar, and you are probably exercising less than you should be. If your diet is rich in sugars and fats, this will tend to raise your blood cholesterol level, and very possibly your blood triglycerides as well. If your lifestyle is sedentary, this will tend to increase your weight, blood pressure, blood fats, and blood sugars, and you will be less able to cope adequately with the stresses of life.

Age, Sex, Heredity

As shown in the preceding list, age has to be considered the most potent risk factor in heart disease. The Framingham Heart Study has shown that simply aging ten years, from 35 to 45 years of age, increases 3.6 times your risk of developing sudden coronary death, myocardial infarction (a "coronary"), and angina pectoris. Going from age 35 to 65 years would increase your risk 8.6 times. Despite its obvious influence, the effect of age is so variable that many people in their eighties, nineties, and even hundreds are apparently free from heart disease and continue to be vigorous to almost the very end of their lives.

Sex is also an important factor. A 45-year-old man, without any other known risk factors, is 3.6 times more likely to develop coronary heart disease than a female of the same age. A 45-year-old female and a 35-year-old male have about the same risk. The risk factors of age and sex are therefore beyond our control because they are part of our God-given destiny.

At first glance it might appear that heredity is also a factor over which we have no control, since studies seem to indicate a real genetic predisposition to heart disease which each of us inherits from our ancestors. The exact nature of this predisposition is not yet entirely clear, although Dr. Glueck, of Cincinnati, has shown that many families in which high numbers of its members live well on into their nineties without heart disease have high levels of HDL (high-density lipoproteins). This apparently allows them to remain free from heart disease, even in spite of higher-than-normal blood-cholesterol levels in some cases. Recent Framingham Heart Study data confirm the benefit of a high level of HDL (more on this later).

Live Right!

While it is true that an ancestral history of heart

disease may predispose you to a heart attack, it is also true that *right living* may actually reduce your probability of suffering heart disease from above average to below average. In other words, even if your family has a history of heart disease, if you are willing to avoid smoking and to maintain your blood pressure and blood cholesterol at proper levels through proper exercise and proper diet, you could reasonably expect to be a *healthier* person than the average population!

The fact that members of your immediate or larger family have had more than their fair share of heart attacks does not *necessarily* mean that you were born with a predisposition to heart disease, since the heart attacks of your family and ancestors could have been caused mostly by wrong living habits.

For example, certain undesirable habits, such as smoking and eating overly rich foods, are often propagated from generation to generation within family groupings. If you have been reared in a family that has been guilty of violating several heart-disease risk factors, then by all means unlearn the bad habits of the past and open the door to vibrant health in your future! Even if you have inherited a bona fide predisposition to heart disease, this tendency can generally be countered by intelligent living habits in your own personal life.

The Lurking Villain

In order to understand clearly why the risk factors

of cigarette smoking, abnormal blood-fat levels, high blood pressure, lack of exercise, mental stress, diabetes, and obesity are so harmful to the health of your heart and body, you must first understand a little about the lurking villain called "atherosclerosis." Atherosclerosis is an extremely common condition among old and young Americans in which cholesterol, a yellowish waxy substance, is deposited on the inside surface of the arteries of the body. In the United States and in many highly civilized Western nations (though seldom in so-called "primitive" nations), atherosclerosis begins in childhood with deposits of fatty streaks on the inside of the body's arteries. These often become more prominent during adolescence and quite pronounced in young adulthood.

Pathologists who performed postmortem examinations of young American soldiers killed during the Korean War were astonished to find that a number of these young men had arteries so completely clogged with cholesterol that only a small opening remained through which blood could pass! And this condition was found in young males who were considered to be in the prime of health!

The Whole Body

Atherosclerosis sometimes involves almost all the arteries of the body, including the arteries of the neck which lead to the brain as well as the arteries which supply blood to the heart muscle (the coronary arteries). Sometimes the major artery from which oxygenated blood flows from the heart to all parts of the body (the aorta) is severely narrowed by atherosclerosis, leading to diminished blood supplies to the chest, abdomen, arms, and legs. Sometimes arteries to the kidneys are involved, or else arteries to the intestines and various vital organs.

Eventually these arteries are not just coated with cholesterol, but they become scarred and inlaid with deposits of fibrous-like materials and calcium. Hemorrhages may occur just beneath the inside surface of the arteries, or clots may form in the remaining narrow opening through which blood flows through the arteries, causing closure. In addition, clots formed elsewhere may be carried by the bloodstream to the narrowed locations and there cause a total blockage (occlusion). If there is narrowing only (but no clots), lack of stamina in various parts of the body can occur. When this kind of narrowing takes place inside the coronary arteries of the heart, there are often symptoms of ''angina pectoris.''

The Angina Warnings

Angina pectoris manifests itself as a sensation of pressure or suffocation in the front of the chest, sometimes accompanied by a feeling of aching numbness of the neck, jaw, or arm. These symptoms are most likely to occur during times of physical or emotional stress, or even after eating a large meal. Angina-triggering physical stress could include work with the arms, or else brisk walking or running (especially uphill), or even being exposed to cold wind. Angina-triggering emotional stress could involve tension, fear, anger, or any variation of these.

The usual treatment for angina pectoris is to place a nitroglycerin pill under the tongue, which usually provides adequate relief within one to five minutes. Some people have frequently recurring symptoms of angina pectoris, especially during times of mental and physical stress, and yet are able to maintain their daily routine without much interruption.

In angina pectoris or any narrowed-artery condition anywhere in the body, the small remaining opening could easily be obstructed by a small amount of bleeding occurring just beneath the inner surface of the artery lining, sometimes even resulting in total obstruction. (Or a clot could form inside the opening of a narrowed artery or be carried there from some other point.) If such an obstruction is nearly complete, and if it occurs within an artery that feeds the heart muscle, a "myocardial infarction" may take place. What this means is that the heart muscle suffers irreversible damage because a number of cells have died. Such a myocardial infarction is popularly referred to as a "heart attack," and in older technical terminology as a "coronary occlusion," or, in shortened form, simply as a "coronary."

The Typical Heart Attack

Although symptoms can vary, the most common symptoms of this kind of "heart attack" include chest pain or pressure, overall physical weakness, nausea, profuse sweating, pain or numbness of the neck, back, abdomen, jaw, shoulders or arms, shortness of breath, irregular heartbeat, and a sense of impending doom. Every year about 600,000 Americans die from coronary heart disease, and as many as 60 percent of these people may die within 24 hours, often very suddenly and with little or no warning.

Sudden death may occur even without any "coronary" or obstruction, and may be related to ischemia (lack of blood flow or oxygen) and electrical instability of the heart. In fact, most resuscitated victims of sudden death have been known to have had marked atherosclerosis or narrowing of the coronary arteries without actually having suffered a myocardial infarction or "coronary."

Various kinds of complications can occur after heart attacks, although modern medical therapy has considerably diminished such complications. Highly trained paramedics, several new miracle drugs, sophisticated electronic monitoring equipment, highly competent doctors and nurses, and a number of other factors have made a heart-attack victim's chances for survival excellent *if he gets treated quickly.* In-hospital mortality for heart attacks has been reduced over a period of years from approximately 30 percent to 15 percent through the use of sophisticated medications and technology, including highly sophisticated coronary care units.

Rehabilitation of heart-attack victims has also progressed enormously, so that with proper medications, and especially physical rehabilitation through exercising, most heart-attack survivors can return to their original occupations within two to four months from the time of their attack.

Measuring the Risks

The basic purpose of this quick survey has been to show that the underlying cause for heart attack (myocardial infarction) is atherosclerosis, or narrowed coronary arteries. By accepted convention, atherosclerosis itself is not included in our list of heart-disease risk factors even though it is of course the major risk factor.

Until recently, atherosclerosis has been considered largely irreversible and usually progressive, being caused by, or at least associated with, the risk factors previously mentioned for heart disease. Recently, however, there has been encouraging news of reversal of atherosclerosis taking place. At least three separate studies involving both rhesus monkeys and humans have demonstrated at least some degree of improvement of previously noted atherosclerosis in some cases.

In the past it has been quite difficult to measure the degree of atherosclerosis-caused narrowing in the arteries of a living person, but now this is being done quite routinely in many medical centers by a pro-

cedure called "coronary angiography" (arterio-
graphy). Recent, more-sophisticated techniques have
been used to demonstrate some evidence of reversal of
atherosclerosis. Many individuals have undergone
angiography for purposes of determining the extent
of atherosclerosis, or narrowing of their coronary
arteries, followed in many cases by surgical bypass of
the blocked arteries with a piece of vein taken from one
of their legs.

This kind of bypass surgery appears to have been of
definite help in many cases of severely blocked
arteries, but the exact role of this kind of surgery in
the management of severe coronary artery disease is
still under hot debate even by specialists. Many
wonder about the widespread use of this expensive,
difficult, and somewhat dangerous procedure. However, most physicians clearly feel that the benefits
outweigh the risks in many situations. Even the coronary angiography itself (the diagnosing procedure)
has a small but definite risk associated with it, and
because of the expense and possible discomfort involved, coronary angiography cannot be carried out
wholesale on everyone.

Stress-testing by use of a treadmill or bicycle
ergometer can also frequently give a clue to the
presence of significant coronary artery disease, particularly when coupled with the new thallium scan-
ning. Even a routine electrocardiogram can give a clue
to the presence of coronary artery disease, sometimes

by suggesting "ischemia" or even the existence of a "scar" of a previously unsuspected or "silent" myocardial infarction.

Atherosclerosis is closely related to several of the other known risk factors, so that when we deal with these factors, we are also closer to dealing with atherosclerosis itself. For example, a person who has high levels of blood cholesterol and blood pressure and who also smokes heavily is very likely to have significant atherosclerosis along with a significant risk of heart attack or stroke.

The Collective Effect

The collective effect of multiple risk factors is staggering. For example, a 45-year-old man with any cigarette smoking at all, with an elevated blood-cholesterol level of 335, with an elevated systolic blood-pressure level of 195, with glucose intolerance short of actual clinical diabetes mellitus, and with some minor abnormalities on his electrocardiogram would have a *16 times higher risk* of sudden death, heart attack, or development of angina pectoris than a 45-year-old man without these same risk factors!

A person who exercises regularly, eats properly, does not smoke, and maintains a normal blood-cholesterol level (especially with associated normal or high HDL) and a normal blood-pressure level is therefore *much* less likely to be afflicted by significant atherosclerosis with its accompanying risk of heart attack and stroke.

A precise relationship between atherosclerosis and every other heart-disease risk factor has not yet been established, even though the overall relationship of these factors (including atherosclerosis) to the heart disease itself has been fairly clearly established. For example, the well-recognized Framingham Heart Study has shown clearly that high blood pressure contributes directly to heart disease. The harmful effects of high blood pressure are so serious that we have devoted much of Chapter 4 to this one risk factor alone.

That Smoke in Your Lungs

How about smoking? Is smoking really harmful to your heart and circulation, or does it just tend to give you lung cancer? The answer is that smoking is extremely harmful to your entire cardiovascular system as well as to your lungs and to all your other major body systems. The Framingham Heart Study shows that the frequent smoking of cigarettes (and to a lesser extent cigars and pipes) contributes very significantly to heart attacks and strokes. There is some question as to whether smoking speeds up the process of atherosclerosis, but there is no question that frequent smoking increases the risk of heart attacks and strokes in people who already have atherosclerosis. Smoking seems to have a particularly profound effect on the incidence of sudden death; any cigarette smoking at all may increase the risk of sudden death by approximately five times.

Smoking of any kind, and especially cigarette smoking, produces profound physiological changes in the human body. The oxygen-carrying capacity of the blood is reduced significantly, and the blood is forced to carry carbon monoxide, a poison which comes from the smoke inhaled into the lungs. Smoking also tends to trigger blood clotting, especially by accelerating the clumping of blood-platelet particles, which become sticky and cling to each other and to the inner walls of the blood vessels. Smoking can also raise the level of blood fats, including cholesterol, which can then become deposited on the inner lining of the arteries. This is further aggravated by the fact that smoking reduces desirably high levels of HDL.

More Problems

In addition, smoking often produces constriction or spasms of the arteries. This decreased blood flow, coupled with the reduction of oxygen and nutrient supply, can seriously threaten the healthful maintenance of various parts of the body. Smokers may notice cool and pale extremities, indicating reduced arterial blood flow as a result of smoking. Smoking can also produce irregularities of the heartbeat (probably by stimulating adrenalin flow), along with increased heartrate, increased blood pressure, and irritation of the heart muscle. This predisposes certain smokers to fatal ventricular fibrillation (nonpumping heart twitchings); in fact, the risk of sudden death for cigarette smokers is between 3 and 17 times higher than for nonsmokers!

The harmful effects of smoking, and especially cigarette smoking, are so serious that cigarette smoking alone, even in the apparent absence of any other known risk factor, can lead to fatal heart attacks. This phenomenon is especially obvious in people under the age of 40. In people over the age of 40, the effects of smoking may be just as harmful as for the younger people, but other risk factors have often built up over the years and tend to work in combination with the negative effects of smoking, thereby making smoking difficult to isolate as the only villain in the case.

This is to say nothing of the chronic lung disease and emphysema with its attendant suffering which may come to people who have been smoking for many years. Chronic lung disease may result in lower oxygen levels in the blood, and may also predispose a person to heart attack. It is clear that the effects of smoking are profound; addiction to cigarette smoking is truly one of the curses of civilization today.

How Do I Stop?

If you are a smoker at present, how do you go about giving up this habit? First, learn the facts about smoking. If you would like more information than we have been able to present in this brief survey, read the literature supplied by the American Heart Association (or other responsible organizations who have research-ed the effects of smoking).

Second, *determine that you will stop smoking.* Smoking is not an easy habit to give up, and you will never relinquish it unless you decide that the job simply must be done. Different methods of discon-tinuing seem to work well for different people, and it is important that you find a method that will work ef-fectively for you. It is beyond the scope of this book to deal with specific smoking-withdrawal methods, but we urge you to make use of whatever help is necessary to discontinue your habit of smoking. If you are a Christian in the born-again definition, you have a sober responsibility before God to maintain your body as "the temple of the Holy Spirit" (1 Corin-thians 6:19,20). However, the good news is that this same Holy Spirit lives inside you in order to give you strength to do what is right.

The Fat Is in Your Blood

The third major villain in the heart-disease epidemic is abnormal blood-fat levels (including high cholesterol levels), as revealed by the Framingham Heart Study and confirmed by other investigations. Cholesterol is a fatty substance which is required in modest amounts in the human body for complete human health, although *excessive* amounts are pro-ven to be extremely harmful. Cholesterol occurs in ex-cessive concentrations in a number of foods, but the main source of cholesterol in the human body is that which is produced by the body itself from saturated fats in the diet. A number of research studies in the U.S. and elsewhere point to the fact that high blood-cholesterol levels are often associated with the development of atherosclerosis as well as with the onset of cardiovascular diseases, such as heart attacks and strokes, as well as angina pectoris.

The effect of high blood-cholesterol levels is particularly insidious because merely lowering the cholesterol levels does not automatically result in a decreased probability of heart disease. This apparent "one-way" effect of deposition of cholesterol on the inner linings of arteries has recently come under closer scrutiny. The potential for at least some degree of reversibility or removal of cholesterol already present is now considered a real possibility. Nevertheless, many scientists have wondered whether the presence of high blood-cholesterol levels is the actual major villain in the present-day epidemic of heart disease.

In my professional judgment, the evidence pointing toward high blood-cholesterol levels as a major villain is so impressive that every adult in America should find what his or her blood-cholesterol level is and should take measures to reduce this level if it is too high.

What Is Normal?

In past years blood-cholesterol levels were con-

sidered normal within a range of 150 milligram percent to 300 milligram percent. However, most car-
diologists and heart-disease researchers now feel that
this range is much too high for optimum health.
Primitive people in areas of the world in which heart
attacks rarely occur invariably have blood-cholesterol
levels far lower than 300 milligram percent, and in
fact usually far lower than 200 milligram percent,
with levels in the range of 120 to 160 being quite
common.

Dr. William Castelli, head of the laboratory used
by the Framingham Heart Study, has found that in
countries in which typical blood-cholesterol levels are
under 150 milligram percent, coronary heart disease is
almost nonexistent. Because of these findings and a
number of others, new maximum-normal levels of
blood cholesterol have been set at about 240 milligram percent, with 150 to 200 now generally considered preferable. These new standards are but-
tressed by evidence that people can have heart attacks
even if their blood-cholesterol levels are only 200 to
250 (apparently because of other risk factors), whereas
people whose blood-cholesterol level is 150 milligram
percent or less almost never suffer heart disease
regardless of other risk factors.

The Lipoproteins

The complex proteins that carry the cholesterol in
the bloodstream (called lipoproteins) are also related

to heart disease. High levels of high-density lipoprotein (HDL) are beneficial to human health, and seem to provide a considerable degree of protection against heart disease. In fact, very recent data indicate that the beneficial effects of high levels of high-density lipoprotein are more important than the level of cholesterol itself. The high-density lipoproteins are so beneficial that they seem to provide significant protection against heart disease even in the presence of relatively high levels of blood cholesterol.

Low-density lipoprotein levels (LDL), on the other hand, seem to aggravate the risk of heart disease when occurring in high levels in the bloodstream. The ideal condition for humans seems to be low blood levels of cholesterol and low-density lipoprotein, and high blood levels of high-density lipoprotein.

Many investigators now believe that the *ratio* of cholesterol levels to HDL levels is the best predictor of coronary heart disease due to blood-fat abnormalities. It is believed that low-density lipoprotein carries cholesterol to the blood vessels, while high-density lipoprotein carries cholesterol from the blood vessels back to the liver, where it is metabolized.

The lipoprotein levels, both high-density and low-density, seem to be at least partly inherited in each individual, although recent studies also seem to indicate that high-density lipoprotein levels can be increased by exercising vigorously (particularly in prolonged aerobic activities, such as running), by giving up smoking, by losing weight, by adopting a prudent diet, and by ingesting small-to-moderate amounts of alcohol. (However, alcohol can pose other serious dangers for some people.)

Before menopause, women have higher levels of high-density lipoproteins than men, and this may be the reason that women are more protected than men against heart attacks, until the time of menopause. Interestingly, men who do long-distance running have high-density lipoprotein levels as high as, if not higher than, women, and would hopefully be similarly protected against coronary heart disease.

The Fats in Your Foods

Total blood-cholesterol levels also respond to diet, and this fact has been well-publicized by recent television ads urging low-cholesterol food substitutes of various kinds. However, one misleading aspect of these ads is that even though a low-cholesterol diet may have *some* beneficial effect on blood-cholesterol levels, *most* cholesterol in the blood does not come from cholesterol in foods at all, but is instead manufactured in the body from saturated fats in the diet. For this reason, the greater emphasis should be placed on reducing the amount of saturated fats that we eat in our foods.

What kinds of foods contain saturated fats? Many "junk foods"—ice cream, most fried foods (including packaged snacks), and virtually all pies and pastries. Other sources of saturated fats include some kinds of meats, particularly beef, lamb, and pork.

35

Chicken, turkey, and fish have exceptionally low levels of saturated fats and are among the most excellent meats available. Eggs contain a fairly high level of cholesterol (though they are an excellent food otherwise), while whole milk and whole-milk products are loaded with saturated fats.

The typical American diet incorporating plenty of beef (including steaks and hamburgers), pork, whole-milk products, eggs, butter, and a whole array of snacky junk foods is grossly overloaded, not only with calories, but also with saturated fats and cholesterol. Americans may get as much as 40 percent of their total calories from saturated fats! This is almost assuredly a significant part of the reason for the epidemic of heart disease in the United States today.

The common U.S. phenomenon of elevated blood triglycerides has also been shown to be somewhat associated with coronary heart disease, although not as dramatically as with blood-cholesterol levels. Triglycerides are manufactured in the human body from carbohydrates, including sugar (and sometimes alcohol). Most Americans would be well-advised to reduce the amount of sugar and alcohol in their diet. Triglyceride levels in the blood also respond well to regular exercise of the proper type, and to weight loss.

The War Survivors

Though a number of studies have been done on low-cholesterol, low-fat, low-sugar diets, none of these studies is more interesting than the observations noted during and after World War Two throughout Europe, especially in the Scandinavian and other northern European countries.

During the war, the people of these countries were compelled to severely restrict their overly-rich food intake, existing instead on a meager supply of vegetables and grain. While this meager diet did have certain undesirable effects, the *overall* effect was one of improved health and increased longevity! Especially striking was the fact that the number of heart attacks and strokes decreased dramatically in spite of the obvious increase in stress caused by the war raging around these people. Postmortem examinations of people dying of various other causes revealed an astonishingly low incidence of atherosclerosis (narrowed arteries). However, within a few years after the war ended, both heart attacks and strokes, as well as postmortem evidence of atherosclerosis, were on the rise again.

A recent Scandinavian study of institutionalized people has shown that blood-fat levels and frequency of coronary heart disease can easily be manipulated upward or downward by simply varying the dietary intake of fat for a few years.

Studies such as these show that a moderate intake of carefully chosen foods can reduce your risk of heart attack and stroke, and can thereby add enjoyable years to your life.

Reversal?

Still other recent studies suggest that atherosclerosis may be reversible, at least to some degree. Studies on rhesus monkeys, as well as special high-quality angiographic X-rays of human leg arteries, have shown that low-cholesterol, low-saturated-fat diets can result in lessening or reversal of narrowing due to atherosclerosis of arteries. Nathan Pritikin, of Southern California, believes that effective exercise combined with a diet containing only 10 percent protein, 10 percent fat, and 80 percent complex carbohydrates (primarily whole grains) is often effective in relieving symptoms of heart disease, and may even help achieve reversal of atherosclerosis.

While cardiovascular diseases are still rampant in the United States, there has been a marked downturn in the occurence of coronary heart disease and stroke since 1968. This has been attributed to a number of factors, including better control of blood pressure and better medical care, especially in the widespread use of coronary care units and in the introduction of new and improved drugs. A significant part of this coronary health improvement has also been produced by beneficial changes in American health habits, including less consumption of saturated fats and of salts, and greater participation in wholesome kinds of exercise. It is clear that great progress can be made in the battle against heart disease when we determine to win this crucial conflict!

3 YOUR HEALTHY HEART

In the previous chapter we discussed the top three factors contributing toward the current epidemic of heart disease in the United States, including age-sex-heredity, cigarette smoking, and abnormal levels of blood fats. In this chapter we would like to consider factors 5 through 9, including lack of exercise, mental stress and Type A personality, diabetes mellitus or glucose intolerance, obesity, and miscellaneous factors (including certain secondary hereditary factors). Factor number 4, high blood pressure, will be reserved for Chapter 4, "Less Is Better."

Although the evidence for the risk factors that we will discuss in this chapter is less dramatic and overwhelming than for the previously-discussed factors of age-sex-heredity, cigarette smoking, and abnormal levels of blood fats, the evidence for these additional factors is nevertheless strongly suggestive, and in some cases quite convincing. With some of these factors, the evidence will probably become totally compelling within the next several years, even as the evidence for cigarette smoking as a major cause of lung cancer moved from the category of highly suggestive to that of totally convincing over a period of 15 to 20 years.

The Scourge of Inactivity

Does a sedentary lifestyle predispose a person to heart disease? Though the answer to this question varies with the researcher, my personal professional judgment after examining numerous research studies is that lack of proper exercise is an extremely important risk factor contributing toward heart disease. In fact, it may very well be that the lack of proper exercise rivals cigarette smoking, abnormal blood-fat levels, and high blood pressure as a major risk factor in heart disease. However, because of the lingering controversy over this issue, I cannot be dogmatic on this point.

The controversy has arisen not because of any lack of studies relating the role of exercise to coronary heart disease, but because of questions asked about the validity and interpretation of these studies. The greatest single criticism of almost all studies in this area has been related to the factor of selection or self-selection of participants in these studies. In other words, perhaps in all these studies the people who were physically active entered such jobs precisely because they were hardier people to begin with; they either selected themselves for this work or perhaps were selected by their employers. Presumably, less robust people would not go into such strenuous lines of work as stevedoring.

Selectivity

A famous example of this phenomenon of selectivity is shown in a 1953 British survey of conductors and drivers of double-decker buses in London. The conductors, who tended to be slender, were rather active on their feet all day, briskly walking back and forth on the aisles and up and down the stairs of their buses; they had a significantly lower rate of heart attack than the drivers, who were sedentary. It was later discovered that the drivers had tended to be heavier than the conductors even at the very outset of their employment, thus showing that some sort of selection process had been going on. This phenomenon of self-selection is of course entirely possible, and perhaps even probable, but in my judgment it fails to explain fully the dramatic difference in longevity and cardiovascular health experienced by the exercising and nonexercising individuals.

To entirely eliminate the self-selection or selected factor by conducting a study in which people who hate exercising are forced to do so would of course be neary impossible, and perhaps even unethical. A completely valid controlled study of the relationship of exercise to heart disease would require many participants, many years of study, a large outlay of money, and perhaps even a totalitarian government

41

to force reluctant people to comply with the testing procedure.

The Positive Results

Nevertheless, some strongly suggestive studies are available which show the beneficial effect of exercise in relation to coronary heart disease. Leon and Blackburn, in a review of about 70 exercise studies, concluded that the positive studies (not all were positive) showed an inverse relationship between activity level and coronary heart disease, with active subjects having one-half the incidence of coronary heart disease and one-third the mortality.

Dr. Ralph Paffenbarger of San Francisco studied longshoremen and noted a definite protective effect (one-third the incidence of sudden death from heart disease) in those workers in the most-active category (those who expended an average of 1876 kilocalories during the ordinary activities of an eight-hour day).

Morris, of England, showed that weekend leisure-time activity for civil-service workers was protective against coronary heart disease if high-intensity exercise levels were reached (7.5 kilocalories per minute or more).

Paffenbarger's latest study, presented to the American Heart Association at Miami Beach in November of 1977, covered nearly 17,000 Harvard alumni and showed that those exercising most vigorously (more than 2000 kilocalories per week beyond ordinary activity levels) cut in half their chances of getting a heart attack. This appeared to be true even in the presence of other coronary risk factors, such as cigarette smoking, age, obesity, high blood pressure, and family history of heart disease. Furthermore, it didn't seem to make any difference if the man had been very active or athletic in college. *Present* vigorous exercise was protective of the alumni regardless of their previous activity level while in college.

The Long-Lived Mountain People

An example of the benefits of vigorous exercise when combined with other wholesome living habits is found among the long-lived citizens of Southern Georgian Russia and of Vilcabamba, Ecuador, as well as among the Hunzas in the Kashmir section of Pakistan. In each of these regions many citizens live beyond the age of 100 years, and some live to be 120 and even older.

My review of several published articles that describe the people from these three locations leads me to believe that daily vigorous physical exercise is probably an important factor contributing to the longevity of these people. All of these people live in mountainous terrain which ranges in altitude from 2000 to 7000 feet, and all of these people are required to walk up and down steep hills and mountains as part of their everyday life schedule. Just to carry out their

43

normal daily activities requires a considerable expenditure of physical energy, and results in a state of remarkable physical fitness for almost all of these citizens regardless of their age.

Of course, other factors may also contribute toward their longevity, such as their low-calorie diet (usually under 2000 calories per day), their low-cholesterol and low-saturated-fat intake (especially in the case of the Ecuadoreans and Hunzas), and their use of wholesome, unrefined foods which are free of chemical preservatives and additives. (For example, whole grains rather than refined flours are used exclusively.)

In addition, there is virtually no air, water, or food pollution, and there is a general sense of satisfying work fulfillment even at the most advanced ages. No one ever retires completely, and close family relationships are maintained throughout the entire life of every person. Also, these three long-lived groups of people live in relatively dry climates that are not buffeted by extreme weather conditions. Heredity could also be involved to some degree, although the long-lived people of southern Georgian Russia are of somewhat mixed stock.

The Measurable Benefits of Exercise

Can any of the benefits of vigorous physical exercise be measured directly by scientific means? Yes. When a person without serious health problems engages regularly in vigorous physical exercise over a period of weeks, the efficiency of his heart is increased, his resting heartrate is reduced (evidencing increased efficiency), the pumping capacity of his heart is increased, his body becomes more efficient in extracting oxygen from the blood, his blood pressure becomes lower, the level of HDL in his blood increases, the level of his serum triglycerides decreases, his serum cholesterol level may drop, and he loses weight—unless, of course, he starts eating more to compensate for his exercising! If the person has been mildly diabetic, his high blood-sugar level may also be reduced.

Nearly every risk factor for coronary heart disease may be beneficially influenced by exercise. Even the desire for cigarette smoking may be curbed or even abolished by aerobic exercise. Since high blood-cholesterol levels, high blood pressure, high blood-sugar levels, and obesity are known heart-disease risk factors, a program of regular, vigorous physical exercise will definitely provide indirect benefit to the health of a person's cardiovascular system.

There is also a possibility (so far not fully established) that regular vigorous exercise continued over a period of years could enlarge the inner diameters of the coronary arteries, thereby providing another means by which heart-attack risk is reduced. Another possible risk-reducing benefit of adequate exercise (not yet fully proven) is the development of supplemental circulation of small blood vessels within the heart ("collateral circulation").

Whether regular vigorous exercise will add years to your life has not yet been proven, but it is surely true that exercise can add life to your years!

The Stresses of Life

The risk factor of life stresses is also significantly related to heart disease. A number of worldwide studies have suggested that incessant, unrelieved stresses of life tend to produce a complex of symptoms which lead to heart disease and other serious ailments. The whole subject of life stresses will be discussed more fully in Chapter 5 of this book, but we should point out here that *some* stresses in daily living are necessary and even wholesome, for stresses stimulate us to do our best in various areas of life. Our goal, in other words, should not be to avoid *all* stresses of life, but simply to avoid *excessive* stresses. Since what is excessive to one person is barely a burden to another, each of us needs to learn his own stress-tolerance limits and to avoid foolhardy ventures into excessively stressful situations.

Doctors Meyer Friedman and Ray Rosenman present the thesis in their book *Type A Behavior and Your Heart* that there are two basic types of human personalities with regard to the issue of stress response. Type B personalities are somewhat relaxed and easygoing and have a lower incidence of heart disease than the general population. Type A personalities are compulsively hard-driving, goal-oriented individuals who never seem to be able to relax adequately. These people have a significantly higher probability of suffering heart disease than the average population. Not everyone is strongly Type A or Type B, but may be more intermediate.

It may even be that the stress-response aspect of personality is partly inherited, and if so, then Type A personalities need to offset their inborn tendency by making well-chosen efforts at relieving excess stress both continuously and at appropriately spaced intervals in their life schedule. The precise thesis of Doctors Friedman and Rosenman is still somewhat controversial, but the general concept that unremitting stress with inadequate release can predispose a person to heart disease is becoming increasingly accepted among medical researchers and physicians.

That Sugar in Your Blood

Another important risk factor that tends to predispose people toward heart disease is diabetes mellitus, a metabolic disorder in which there is inadequate insulin, resulting in excess glucose sugar appearing in the blood and sometimes even in the urine. Even people with mildly elevated blood-sugar levels seem to have a much greater disposition to atherosclerosis as well as to premature heart attack and stroke. Diabetes of this type may be hereditary, but it can also be acquired partly by improper diet and development of obesity, and perhaps also by other wrong living habits.

Overweight people, especially those who have a high intake of refined carbohydrates (such as sugar) are much more likely to have diabetes than people of normal weight and temperate dietary habits. In fact, many physicians now believe that people who hold their weight within normal levels and avoid highly refined carbohydrates (eating instead complex carbohydrates such as those found in whole, unrefined grains) are not likely to develop the most common form of diabetes even if their hereditary background is less than ideal. It has recently been clearly demonstrated that blood-sugar levels of diabetic people can be lowered by the simple addition of bran to their diet. There is also some evidence that a long-term dietary deficiency of chromium (and perhaps other trace minerals and vital food elements) may also predispose a person to diabetes mellitus. The comments in this paragraph apply particularly to diabetes which begins in adulthood, since diabetes which begins in childhood or young adulthood may be much more closely associated with inherited characteristics and perhaps even viral illnesses (rather than with wrong diet or poor living habits).

The Side-Effects of Overweight

Significant overweight is also a heart-disease risk factor, although somewhat indirectly. The Framingham Heart Study showed that even though obesity all by itself is not a direct risk factor of heart disease, obesity does tend to aggravate other risk factors which are clearly related to heart disease. For example, a person who is 20 percent or more overweight is much more likely than a normal-weight person to have high blood pressure, high blood cholesterol, and diabetes, each of which is an important risk factor related to heart disease. Also, significant overweight is usually tangible evidence that a person has not been engaging in regular, vigorous physical exercise! We will deal with the issue of losing weight in Chapter 7.

The Other Factors

As we mentioned previously, incorrect diet is an indirect heart-disease risk factor in that the wrong choice of foods and the overindulgence in food often leads to high blood pressure, high blood cholesterol, and diabetes, all three of which are extremely significant risk factors. There may also be other diet-related risk factors whose relationship to heart disease has not yet been clearly established. For example, people with elevated blood-uric-acid levels also appear to have a somewhat higher risk of heart disease, although this is thought by most medical scientists to not actually have a causative role in heart disease, but to be merely an association.

Some researchers feel strongly that the heavy use of refined white sugar (sucrose) contributes significantly to heart disease. Other researchers feel that inadequate intake of Vitamin C can make the arteries more susceptible to atherosclerosis. Some evidence seems to point to a relationship between inadequate magnesium intake (and certain other minerals naturally occurring in hard water) and increased incidence of heart disease, while other evidence suggests that a deficiency of Vitamin B-6 or even of Vitamin E could possibly also have similar effects.

A number of other dietary correlations have been proposed (trace minerals in the diet, chlorinated water, bleached flour, etc.), but some aspects of nutritional research with respect to heart disease are in a state of comparative infancy. The coming months and years will in all probability provide additional important correlations between nutrition and cardiovascular well-being.

Puffing and the Pill

There is another heart-disease risk factor which is of particular interest to childbearing women and their families, and that is the use of birth-control pills. For women who do not smoke, the use of birth-control pills increases the risk of heart attack moderately, but in women who *do* smoke and who also use birth-control pills, the risk of heart attack is increased dramatically. (For younger women who do not smoke, but do use birth-control pills, there is only a very slight increase in heart-attack probability.) And of course smoking alone significantly increases the probability of heart disease for any adult, as we emphasized in the previous chapter.

Inherited Risk?

In the previous chapter we mentioned the risk factor of heredity in heart disease, and we should reiterate here that in most cases the hereditary predisposition toward the most common form of heart disease (arteriosclerotic) can be more than offset by the intelligent application of right living habits. This does not necessarily apply to other forms of heart disease, such as those of rheumatic or congenital origin. However, even these can be aided by right living habits, and sometimes these forms of heart disease respond dramatically to today's sophisticated new medical and surgical techniques.

Sometimes what is thought to be an inherited tendency toward heart disease is nothing but an acquired tendency toward bad living habits. Altogether too many parents, grandparents, aunts, and uncles teach growing children by their own bad example that the overconsumption of fatty, sugary, snacky foods is an acceptable part of daily living. Sometimes this negative example extends to heavy liquor consumption and heavy smoking as well, along with little or no physical exercise and inadequate release of tensions. No wonder children grow up predisposed to heart disease and a dozen other ailments!

You Can Do It!

At first the interrelationship of the various heart-disease risk factors may seem overwhelmingly complicated, but actually it is not all that difficult to eliminate or at least significantly reduce almost all of these risk factors in your own life. For example, if you avoid smoking, exercise regularly and vigorously, cope adequately with daily stresses, eat a balanced diet of wholesome foods in moderate quantities, and reduce your weight to normal (or preferably slightly below normal), you will have directly or indirectly reduced or eliminated most of the heart-disease risk factors which are known to medical science at this date. Some individuals may need to take prescribed medication under the supervision of a physican in order to reduce the levels of their blood pressure, blood sugar, or blood fats, but in most cases prescription medications will not be necessary if a person follows an intelligent program of proper diet, adequate exercise, and effective relaxation.

4 LESS IS BETTER

"Don't get so excited! Remember your high blood pressure!" Although these half-jesting words have been spoken to many a harried businessman, the sad fact is that they could just as well be spoken to millions of other Americans, for reliable surveys show that as many as 25 million Americans have some degree of high blood pressure, many of them unknowningly.

High blood pressure, technically called hypertension, is such a widespread malady that it affects not only older people but also young and middle-aged adults in the prime of life and in their most productive years. High blood pressure is sometimes even found in children, although it most often begins in the thirties and increases gradually throughout life. Very often death is caused directly or indirectly by high blood pressure, especially death by strokes and coronary heart disease. The shocking fact is that 35 to 40 percent of all people 60 years of age or older in the United States today have at least some degree of high blood pressure!

Measuring Your Pressure

As most people are aware, blood pressure is usually measured with a gauge and hose connected to a cloth cuff which is wrapped around a person's arm. The doctor or nurse who does the measuring also uses a stethoscope to listen to the blood-pressure sounds in the arm at the inner bend of the elbow so that he or she can know exactly when to note the blood-pressure values indicated on the gauge.

Blood-pressure values are usually indicated in millimeters of mercury and are considered normal for adults up to a maximum reading of 140 over 90. The upper or first number is the "systolic" pressure and refers to the pressure generated by the heart as it pumps blood into the arteries. The lower or second number is the "diastolic" pressure and refers to the pressure that exists in the arteries between beats of the heart. This value is related to the internal diameter of the arteries, which in turn is related to the arteries' condition of tension or contraction.

Both the systolic (upper) and diastolic (lower) pressures are important, and a high reading in either of these two pressures is now considered equally serious, especially if the readings are significantly above 140 over 90. The World Health Organization considers any reading equal to or greater than 160 over 95 to constitute significant high blood pressure. A national health survey conducted by the Public Health Service shows that about 15 percent of all whites and 28 percent of all blacks have high blood pressure by this definition.

In general, the higher the blood pressure, the more serious its effects, especially if the hypertension continues for a number of years. Some people have moderate high blood pressure only occasionally (called "labile" hypertension), but even these occasional elevations result in some increase in the risk of serious cardiovascular diseases later in life. Many people who have only mild or intermittent high blood pressure in their youth develop continuous high blood pressure in the later years of their life. Very recently, some investigators have expressed the view that most hypertension begins in childhood or even infancy with blood-pressure levels that are only slightly higher than those of their peers, but still within limits that have traditionally been accepted as normal.

The Effects of Hypertension

High blood pressure has a number of serious effects in the human body, since virtually all of the body is fed by blood flowing through arteries. High blood pressure causes the muscular coats around the arteries to be in a continual state of "spasm" or excessive tension, thereby narrowing the passageways through which the blood flows. Eventually the artery walls become permanently thickened or "hypertrophied," making the narrowed passageways a more permanent feature of high blood pressure.

Hypertension also increases significantly your probability of suffering a stroke, because the arteries which lead to the head and brain are directly affected by high blood pressure. If an artery in or near the brain bursts (sometimes at the point of a bubble or "aneurism" in an artery), it can flood critical areas of the brain with blood and lead to unconsciousness, brain damage, and death.

Long-term high blood pressure often results in damage to the heart: as the heart pumps month after month and year after year at a too-high pressure against an increased resistance, the walls of the heart tend to become thickened ("hypertrophied"), and eventually the heart becomes enlarged ("dilated"), eventually leading to congestive heart failure. Chest X-rays of people with long-term high blood pressure often show pathological enlargement of the heart, and electrocardiograms often reveal abnormal patterns caused by such enlargement.

Prolonged high blood pressure often reduces the blood flow in the kidneys, leading to progressive damage and decreased ability to rid the bloodstream of waste products. Sometimes total kidney failure results. Even your eyes can be affected by high blood pressure, since the arteries of the eyes are extremely sensitive to abnormalities of any kind. Since the arteries of the eyes are the only arteries in the human body that can be adequately examined in living people, physicians often use a viewing device called an ophthalmoscope to examine the condition of the arteries within the eyes, thereby gaining important clues to the damage done by hypertension in the rest of the body.

High blood pressure also tends to accelerate the process of atherosclerosis, in which blood fats are deposited on the inside of the arteries. As we mentioned earlier, such fat deposits result in narrowed passageways for the blood and an increase likelihood of blood clotting, strokes, coronary heart disease, and a whole host of related ailments.

Why So High?

If the silent menace of high blood pressure is such a villain in the human body, exactly what is it that causes such hypertension? In a minority of cases (perhaps 5 to 15 percent) the exact cause can be pinpointed, although in most cases the exact cause is extremely hard to prove conclusively. Proven causes of high blood pressure include kidney disease (the reverse phenomenon can also take place—high blood pressure from other causes can induce kidney failure), physical damage of the kidneys or their arteries, adrenal disease of various kinds, excessive thyroid activity, a narrowing of the major heart artery (the aorta), pregnancy, ovarian tumors, lead and cadmium poisoning, ingestion of certain cheeses or licorice candy, high blood calcium, and oral contraceptives ("the pill").

Hard-to-prove causes of high blood pressure include fear, anger, or life stresses in general, long suspected as villains. It is definitely known that such emotions may temporarily raise blood pressure through the secretion of such hormones as adrenalin and noradrenalin, but the question is whether such emotions can *permanently* elevate blood-pressure levels. Many scientists now believe that, for some people who are exposed to unremitting stresses of life with no adequate release, the continuing secretion of these hormones (and perhaps others) does indeed produce high blood pressure with all its vicious side effects.

Heredity may also play some part in high blood pressure, but probably not to the extent that hypertension is inevitable for any given person. In other words, proper living habits can likely prevent blood-pressure levels from rising above normal even for those people who have a hereditary predisposition toward hypertension.

The Salt Monster

There is also considerable evidence that excessive intake of ordinary salt (sodium chloride) may contribute significantly to high blood pressure. There is general agreement among most researchers and physicians that people in the United States (and Western civilization generally) consume far too much salt. Studies have shown that in those societies (usually primitive ones) in which salt consumption is very low (less than two grams of sodium per day), high blood pressure is virtually nonexistent. However, when these people become "civilized" with Western diets and living habits, they start to suffer high blood pressure and most of the other deadly diseases of Westen civilization!

Actually, you may be consuming a large amount of salt without even realizing it, since in all probability your greatest ingestion of salt does not come directly from a saltshaker at all. If you are a typical American, you consume large amounts of "hidden" salt in the form of packaged foods of every description. The great majority of all foods eaten in the United States today (including virtually all "junk foods") are heavily flavored with salt and various other sodium-laden additives.

Those physicians who specialize in treating high blood pressure are so convinced of the harmful effects of excessive salt intake that they are virtually unanimous in recommending restricted salt intake as a first step in treatment. Often they also prescribe diuretics for their patients in order to accelerate the excretion of sodium chloride through the kidneys. In many cases of mild or early high blood bressure, salt restriction alone, with no medications, or perhaps minimal medications, is successful in restoring normal blood pressure.

Although a really sophisticated salt-restriction diet requires the personal counsel of a qualified physician and perhaps even a dietitian, a good starting point is to eliminate as much as possible all foods that are obviously salty, and with your physician's permission replace the common table salt in your saltshaker with one of the several potassium chloride substitutes available today. (Fifty-fifty blends of sodium chloride and potassium chloride are now also available in the supermarkets.)

The American Heart Association and other organizations have published extensive listings of the salt content in various foods, and here is a brief rundown of the worst offenders:

French fries, pretzels, potato chips
sauerkraut
pickles
corned beef
sausages
frankfurters
cured ham
canned fish
frozen oysters
green olives
waffles
most cheeses
most canned and dried soups
most canned vegetables
many breads and cereals

At first the thought of decreasing your salt intake may seem impossible because of your love of salt-laden foods, but the experience of many thousands of people has proven the fact that you can actually learn to decrease your craving for such foods within a few weeks of improved eating habits.

Another way of dealing with the problem of excessive salt in your body is to simply sweat it out! Vigorous physical exercise (assuming that you are safely able to do it) can be an effective means of excreting excess salt. A hot environment (whether in a sauna room or else-where) also induces sweating and salt excretion, although excessive heat also tends to produce various health problems in a significant number of people.

Many other factors, including excessive cadmium intake (from smoking, from a polluted environment, and from refined foods) have been proposed as causes contributing to high blood pressure. Much more research needs to be done on these various contributing causes, but is certainly safe to say that a diet which rejects highly processed and refined foods in favor of whole and unrefined ones is a right step in the direction of overall health.

Know Your Pressure

How do you know if you have high blood pressure? If you are middle-aged or older, and if your blood pressure has been high for a number of years, you may be experiencing some of the symptoms described earlier in this chapter. However, in the majority of cases high blood pressure is truly a silent menace, because its symptoms are not particularly noticeable until after they have already done significant damage in your body, sometimes even irreversible damage. *It is therefore critically important that every adult have regular medical checkups which include blood-pressure evaluation.*

If your blood-pressure reading on your first visit seems high, one or more subsequent visits may be necessary in order to determine the dynamics of the blood pressure in your body (since blood pressures can vary significantly from day to day and even from minute to minute). Be sure to visit one of the many physicians who are aware of the most recent consensus on safe blood-pressure values.

In past years it was thought that a safe upper (systolic) blood-pressure reading could be as high as 100 plus a person's age. In other words, a 60-year-old person could safely have an upper reading of 160 millimeters of mercury. However, recent research has shown this older view to be clearly erroneous, and most doctors who specialize in the treatment of high blood pressure today feel that readings should never remain higher than 140 over 90 regardless of age, and should ideally be somewhat lower than these numbers. In the words of the National Conference of High Blood Pressure Education, "Hypertensive disease is a massive public health problem in the United States—one of the most important, if not *the* most important, affliction producing premature sickness, disability, and death in our adult population" *(Report of Proceedings,* January 15, 1973).

Getting Those Numbers Down

If your blood pressure is only slightly high, your physician will probably ask you to restrict your salt intake, to make better arrangements for dealing with your life stresses, to lose weight, and perhaps to begin a sensible program of physical exercise. If your blood pressure is significantly higher than normal, your doctor will probably prescribe diuretic pills in order to help your body rid itself of excess salt. He may also prescribe medications which will help increase the inner diameter of your arteries, thereby allowing the blood to flow more easily and also reducing your blood pressure.

After your blood pressure has been reduced to safe levels by these means, your doctor may very likely prescribe a controlled physical exercise program which can help to reduce your blood pressure still further. (Mounting evidence shows that weight loss is considerably more effective than previously realized in reducing both systolic and diastolic blood pressure.) Some people are able to discontinue blood-pressure medications altogether through a combination of restricted salt intake, loss of weight, regular physical exercise, and decreased life stresses (if possible). However, people who have high blood pressure should realize that the treatment of hypertension, whether requiring prescribed medications or not, should be considered a lifelong matter.

Regular exercise which is physically vigorous is so helpful in maintaining normal blood pressure and in stimulating your general physical health that everyone who is physically able to do it should exercise vigorously and intelligently at least three times a week. (However, if you have not had a medical checkup lately, be sure to get one before you begin any exercise program, since significant high blood pressure, or any one of several other ailments, requires special considerations before beginning any physical exercise program.)

We will be devoting all of Chapter 6 to the joys and rewards of physical exercise, but we need to say here that regular exercise of the vigorous "aerobic" kind is now known to lower overall blood pressure (both upper and lower readings). In a healthy person, the *immediate* effect of vigorous exercise is to lower his diastolic pressure and raise his systolic pressure, but for most people the *long-term* effect of vigorous exercise is to reduce both figures.

When your blood pressure comes down, well-established statistics show that you reduce your likelihood of suffering congestive heart failure, stroke, kidney failure, and several other related ailments. With today's medical knowledge about control of high blood pressure, there is really no reason for anyone to put up with the continuing hazards of this deadly lurking menace.

5 POWER OVER PRESSURE

"Howard! I need that report before five o'clock this afternoon!" This had been a typical business demand placed on Howard in the days and weeks before his heart attack. The boss was not cruel, but he simply needed a tremendous amount of accurate information prepared in a minimum of time.

In order to provide this information, Howard needed the help of two secretaries, eight engineers and lab technicians, one computer programmer, one comptroller, three service representatives, and five on-the-road sales representatives. Added to his own struggle to avoid errors in judgment as a middle-level executive, Howard had to deal with the daily problems of 20 subordinates, including informational errors, judgmental errors, absenteeism, and occasional personality conflicts.

The job seemed almost too much at times, but it did pay well, and there was realistic hope of considerable future advancement. Added to Howard's work responsibilities were his family responsibilities toward Lois and the two children. And then there was the weekly yardwork, car maintenance, and remodeling of the garage. Sometimes Howard wondered how he could handle the total responsibilities of his life without just collapsing.

Lois was not exactly idle, either. She was the mother of two active children, one of them a teenager, and she worked 30 hours a week as a teacher's aide at a local junior high school. In addition, she headed two women's groups at church, and still found time to keep her house close to immaculate! For Lois as well as for Howard, the pressures of life sometimes seemed simply overwhelming.

Is This Your Life?

Does any of this sound familiar to you? It should, because millions of Americans are going through this kind of pressure cooker every day of their lives! Is this pressure killing us, or is it just spurring us on to higher and better accomplishments?

The answer is that it is doing both of these things. A certain amount of pressure in life is wholesome to the extent that is stimulates us to do our best both physically and mentally. For example, the pressure of a competitive economic system has stimulated the American people to become highly efficient in producing a vast array of useful and enjoyable goods and services. Communist countries that lack such a competitive economic system are simply no match for the United States (and other Western democratic nations) when it comes to producing high-quality goods and services. The principle of competitive pressure also applies quite dramatically in the whole realm of sports. The challenge of besting another team or individual spurs people on to record-breaking accomplishments.

Those Deadly Stresses

On the other hand, *too much* physical or mental stress is deadly. Firemen in the large cities of the United States have among the highest heart-attack rates of any occupational group in the world, and many researchers believe that this high rate is caused by the intense physical and emotional stress which these firemen undergo intermittently in an otherwise-sedentary life.

But you don't need to be a fireman in order to abuse your body with the serious effects of long-term overstress. A number of years ago Dr. Walter B. Cannon described the basic defense-alarm reaction or fight-flight response that occurs when animals or people are faced with stressful situations. In general, the emotion of either anger or fear (or both) results in a desire to either fight or flee. In these situations, a person's blood pressure and pulse-rate often rise dramatically for a period of minutes or even hours.

Your Stress Reactions

A number of scientists feel that the present epidemic of high blood pressure in modern Western society is caused at least partially by frequent stressful situations of various kinds with very little opportunity for adequate release of stress between each situation. In 1956, Dr. Hans Selye, one of the world's leading authorities on stress, published *The Stress of Life,* in which he outlined three basic stages which human beings experience in response to various kinds of severe emotional stress.

First there is a reaction of alarm; then there is resistance (an ability to meet that particular stress successfully as a result of adaptation); finally there is an inner exhaustion which leads to an almost-total depletion of energy reserve. In many cases this exhaustion is both physical and psychological (and sometimes spiritual as well) because of the complex interworking of the entire human personality.

Often-repeated stress without adequate opportunity for release probably increases the likelihood not only of stroke but also of fatal and near-fatal heart attacks, as well as of several other diseases. Dr. Richard Rahe, a psychiatrist, has published clinical studies that identify prolonged stress with just such diseases. His analysis of various stressful events of life seems to indicate that in many cases major illnesses follow severe stresses within a matter of weeks or months. A recently concluded 40-year study of Boston college students has clearly demonstrated that those students who had better mental health also enjoyed better physical health, with fewer diseases in the ensuing years.

The Frustrated Specialists

At the time the U.S. space program was being severely curtailed in the early 1970's, there began a rash of fatal and near-fatal heart attacks on the part of the scientists and other highly skilled personnel at Cape Canaveral (Cape Kennedy). These men and women knew that they would soon be losing their employment at the Space Center, but would find little opportunity to continue to use their skills elsewhere in the United States, or anyplace else in the world, for that matter. They were in a highly frustrating, no-win situation and were experiencing the effects of a long "fight-and-flight" reaction with a chronic state of "visceral-vascular readiness." There was simply no way of adequately releasing their stressful frustrations, and a significant percentage of these people experienced a common end product—fatal and near-fatal heart attacks.

When pathologist Dr. Robert Elliott was called upon to investigate this high incidence of heart attacks and sudden deaths at Cape Canaveral, his postmortem examinations uncovered a most unusual phenomenon. Instead of finding typical curvy fibers upon microscopic examination of the heart muscle (the kind of fibers often found in a heart attack attributable to atherosclerosis), he found unusual "contraction bands" of the heart muscle, with less-than-expected atherosclerosis of the coronary arteries. Since that time these "contraction bands" have been correlated with stress and a high secretion of certain body hormones, such as adrenalin and noradrenalin.

Fight or Run?

If stress is so harmful, what can we do about it? Should we simply run away from it, or should we try to face it? If we are trying to face a tremendous load of stresses in our lives but seem to be losing the battle, what can we do about it? A large number of people, including college students, elderly sick people, and even middle-aged professionals, seem to think that suicide is the only answer, but certainly there is a better response than this.

The first thing we need to recognize is that we do not want to eliminate all stresses in our lives. As we indicated earlier in this chapter, a certain amount of stress is highly desirable in order to stimulate us to be at our best spiritually, psychologically, and physically. We also need to remember that people vary widely in their capacity to endure or even enjoy the usual stresses of life. To one person, real-estate selling may be an enjoyable, stimulating challenge, while to another person the same occupation may be an overwhelming burden of time and energy.

For this reason it is critically important that each one of us learn the kind of stresses that we are able to handle best, and then live within the framework of these kinds of daily stresses as much as possible. This is really not as hypothetical as it may sound, since many of us do have at least some control over the kinds of life situations in which we live.

Talk About Your Problems

For example, for many people it is realistically possible to change jobs or at least to modify certain responsibilities within a continuing job. Since a new job often brings pressures and pitfalls which have not been anticipated, many people would be wise to first pursue the possibilities of making necessary changes in their present job. Many thousands of employees would be surprised to find how responsive their employers can be if they receive requests for changes which are reasonable and which are presented courteously.

This kind of reasonable and courteous communication is particularly fruitful in reducing tensions and pressures in husband-wife relationships. Sometimes there is a fine line between a legitimate retreat from overbearing pressures and a cowardly escape from legitimate responsibilities, but frank and courteous discussion between the parties involved can in a surprising number of cases resolve this issue to everyone's satisfaction.

Our Attitudes Toward Stress

Since most of us are faced with various heavy life stresses from time to time no matter how wisely we may try to arrange our life situation, and since others of us seem to face heavy stresses practically every day of our lives, we all need to know how to cope effectively with stresses.

If we are born-again Christians, we need to recognize that our ultimate strength for facing the stresses of life comes from God Himself, and if we are not born-again Christians we need to recognize the fact that accepting help from heaven is not a cowardly escapist technique at all, but is a legitimate attitude of life which God approves of and even expects from everyone. If we can recognize that, like Job, each of us is expected to carry a certain measure of burdens not caused by our own shortcomings, then we will learn to accept the pressure-producing people in our lives with spiritual maturity rather than with shortsighted resentment.

For some people, excessive self-perfectionism greatly increases the total burden of pressure in their lives. While perfectionism can be put to useful purposes and is in fact a vital part of any civilized society, every perfectionist needs to learn to *control* his perfectionism so that it does not possess him in every activity of life. A perfectionist who has not learned this kind of control is often haunted by feelings of guilt because of the minor shortcomings he sees in his career and in his various other activities of life.

But how about those of us who simply must face various kinds of pressures every day of our lives? How can we adequately cope with such pressures? In addition to adopting proper attitudes toward such pressures, as we mentioned previously, each of us needs to get adequate and regular release from such pressures. Legitimate release from pressures is not only a proper activity of life, but it is absolutely essential to normal health and sanity.

The Illegitimate Releases

Before discussing specific ways to find legitimate release from the pressures of life, let us briefly consider some illegitimate releases. These include such defeatist escape techniques as the use of illegal drugs or excessive alcohol, illegitimate absenteeism from work, reckless driving, desertion from family and employment responsibilities, or even suicide.

As most of you are well aware, illegal drugs of many kinds are now being used in epidemic proportions in the United States. Almost all of these are harmful to the body in one or more ways, with some of them producing irreparable damage. Even marijuana, which is considered the least harmful of the illegal or quasilegal drugs, may produce subtle personality changes after prolonged use, as well as possible damage to human genes and offspring.

Alcoholism is another escapist epidemic that is afflicting the United States down to ages as low as the teen years or even lower. Even though the use of alcohol is legal for adults, its damage to the body can be truly devastating. Not just the liver, but the brain and entire human metabolism can be severely damaged by the excessive use of alcohol. Because of the physically damaging effects of both alcohol and illegal drugs, these two escapist techniques are not really escapes at all, since the drug or alcohol addict is caught in a descending spiral of deteriorating health which reduces his ability to handle any of the normal pressures of life and eventually leads to serious disease and premature death.

Illegitimate absenteeism also has reached epic proportions in the United States, with hundreds of millions of dollars worth of employment services lost annually. While it is true that overwork can indeed be a source of serious overpressure, illegitimate absenteeism is certainly not the answer, since it increases tensions between employer and employee and in the final analysis adds to rather than substracts from the total amount of pressure in the employee's life.

Hostile or reckless driving is a serious problem on the highways of the United States, according to police reports from most states in the country. Careful police investigations reveal that time after time a driver who caused a serious or fatal accident had just engaged in a heated argument with his or her spouse or employer.

And of course alcoholism is also heavily involved in the entire incompetent-driving syndrome, since approximately 50 percent of all fatal automobile accidents in the United States involved at least one driver who had been drinking.

Desertion of family or employer might at first seem like a rare, last-ditch effort at escaping excess pressures, but actually many thousands of adults desert their family and employment each year in the United States. In some ways this is the most pathetic form of escape of all, since the person who runs away not only leaves behind heartbreak and turmoil, but also usually establishes a new set of knotty problems for himself and others in his new location.

If you have been tempted to retreat into one of these false havens of escape, read on and consider the following *legitimate* methods of escaping the pressures of life.

The Need for Sleep

First of all, get adequate sleep. This may seem like an overly obvious statement, but actually millions of Americans have not had an adequate night of sleep in many months or years. Many people are caught in a tyrannical treadmill of frenetic activities until midnight or beyond, only to have to rise at 6:00 or 6:30 in order to be able to make it to work on time. In some cases these poor sleep habits begin in the pressure of college days, while in other cases these habits develop out of the pressures of an overly busy professional career.

But whether for these reasons or others, the habit of staying busy until midnight and then being compelled to rise fairly early in the morning keeps the body in a continual state of partial sleep deprivation. While it is true that a few people seem to get along quite well with only four to six hours of sleep a night, most people need seven to nine hours each night in order to be fully rested and vigorous. For some people, even this much sleep is not enough because they are suffering from a general lack of physical fitness or from some other specific ailment.

However, there is another large group of Americans who would gladly sleep eight or nine hours a night and would be more than willing to schedule their time to do this, but who simply cannot sleep more than four or five hours during any given night no matter how they schedule their time. This kind of partial insomnia is a tremendous problem in the United States, as evidenced by the barrage of sleeping-pill ads that we see on TV.

(Too much sleep can also be harmful. A recent study showed that people who regularly sleep more than ten hours a night have an increased risk of death due to coronary heart disease, even as do those people who regularly sleep less than five hours a night.)

The Pros and Cons of Pill-Popping

What is the answer for such people who cannot

sleep properly? Since adequate sleep is such a critically important part of overall good health, every person with a significant sleeplessness problem should do everything in his or her power to correct this situation. If the sleeplessness occurs only occasionally, sleeping pills *may* provide some worthwhile help. However, nonprescription sleeping pills tend to produce drowsiness rather than real sleep, and when sleep does come it is often accompanied by abnormal dream patterns. Also, some brands of nonprescription sleeping pills are toxic in high doses and tend to be habit-forming.

Prescription sleeping pills are somewhat more effective, but these also tend to inhibit normal dream patterns (which are a necessary means of subconscious release of pressure). In addition, their effect tends to wear off after a few days or weeks, requiring even larger doses to produce any sleep at all. There are some truly effective prescription sedations available, but unfortunately these tend to be strongly addictive and produce various undesirable side effects.

For many people, a more effective short-term remedy for sleeplessness is found in one of the various kinds of prescription "minor" tranquilizers, though some people find such "minor" tranquilizers ineffective or else find that they produce undesirable side effects. Nevertheless, prescription "minor" tranquilizers are usually to be preferred over sleeping pills because they are more relaxing, they do not seriously inhibit dreams, they remain reasonably effective even after continued use, and in most cases they are not habit-forming. However, even prescription "minor" tranquilizers should be considered a temporary rather than a permanent aid to proper sleep. (Certain people with special physical or mental problems may need to use certain kinds of tranquilizers on a long-term basis.)

Walk Yourself to Sleep

For most people, a much better alternative to sleeping pills or tranquilizers as an aid to restful sleep (except for temporary use as described above) is adequate physical exercise. Various studies have shown that physical exercise of a relaxing nature such as brisk walking, jogging, bicycling, swimming, etc., tends to be even more effective than prescription tranquilizers in providing restful and adequate sleep for people with sleeping problems. This kind of exercise is most effective in aiding sleep when it is performed several hours before bedtime. (However, for some people walking is about equally effective as a relaxant whether performed just before bedtime or a few hours sooner.)

In our American system, only products or services that produce a profit are advertised on TV, and that is why sleeping pills rather than exercise are touted as the cure-all for insomnia. But if you want a low-cost, wholesome, and effective method of sleeping tonight, try some reasonably vigorous physical exercise from one to four hours before your normal bedtime!

Actually, vigorous physical exercise may do more than help you get a good night's rest—it may provide the mental and physical relaxation you need in order to put up with the pressures and stresses in your life. Many joggers experience a sense of complete relaxation after covering a few miles at an easy pace at the end of a long, hard day. A program of regular vigorous aerobic exercise may not only help in dealing with the stresses and problems of that particular day, but it could and should be part of a regular program to deal with stress on a long-term basis.

How to Withdraw and What to Drink

One sleep-inducing technique which many people find very effective is that of "gradual withdrawal," in which they avoid all mentally challenging or emotionally upsetting activities during the last two or three hours of the evening before bedtime. This is actually a very legitimate kind of escape technique, since it often enables a person to face the new challenges of the next day with much greater vigor than if he or she had tossed and turned sleepless for the first two or three hours of the night. Many people find that quiet music, relaxing reading, or an enjoyable hobby can be an important part of this kind of gradual-withdrawal technique.

Of course there are also many other techniques which people use in order to find sleep at night. Since each person has certain individualities about him, it could easily be that one person's special technique for sleeping at night could work effectively for him or her even though it seems to be of little value to the general public. Drinking a glass of warm milk just before bedtime seems to be helpful to quite a few people, apparently because of the amino acid *tryptophane* which is present in the milk.

Another extremely effective method of finding rest at night, especially for born-again Christians, is that of prayer to God and quiet reading in selected passages of the Bible. Even in the midst of severe persecution, David of the Old Testament could say, "I laid me down and slept . . . for the Lord sustained me" (Psalm 3:5). Even in our technological twentieth century, the psalms of the Old Testament provide extremely effective assurance and peace.

Getting Away From It All

How else can we get effective relief from the inevitable pressures of life? By taking daily, weekly, and yearly vacations. By daily vacations, we mean that everyone should spend at least one hour every day in some kind of activity that he finds enjoyable and relaxing. If this enjoyable activity includes vigorous physical exercise, so much the better, since this will benefit a person in far more ways than just releasing the pressures of life. As we mentioned in the previous section on insomnia, activities which many people find both enjoyable and relaxing include music, reading, hobbies, and many other varieties of activities.

By weekly vacations, we mean that no one should work seven days a week on a regular basis; everyone should enjoy at least one day a week that is free from heavy work pressures. Of course, we recognize that under certain conditions some people are compelled to work seven days during certain given weeks, but our point is that this seven-workdays-a-week routine often leads to physical illness if continued for a period of weeks or months.

It is also a good idea to take weekend vacations away from home several times a year. Even people who must live on limited budgets find that they are able to do this if they plan ahead wisely. As families get involved in these weekend vacations, they find choice opportunities to build up family ties that tend to get frayed during the frenetic pressure of the modern American family's daily grind.

How about yearly vacations? Theoretically, these are not absolutely essential if a person or family maintains a proper schedule of daily or weekly vacations, with several weekend trips away from home every year. However, most individuals and families seem to find that a one-to-three-week vacation every year provides tremendous enjoyment and relaxation.

Pressured Relaxation?

Earlier in this chapter we mentioned that hobbies can be an effective and legitimate means of temporarily escaping from the pressures of life. At this point, we should mention one important qualification to this statement: hobbies are truly relaxing *only if they are devoid of intense pressures of their own.* For example, many men who play golf actually compete more fiercely in this game than they do in the business world. If you feel that you simply *must* reduce your golf score to the low seventies, you may actually be adding another unnecessary pressure to your life instead of escaping from the excess pressures that you already have!

The same can be true of many other hobbies, especially if the participant is a Type A personality (a hard-driving, compulsive perfectionist). People who tend to manufacture their own stresses in their hobbies need to become aware of this fact and to counter it by changing their attitude toward their hobbies or else by changing the hobbies themselves.

Food and Your Nerves

Proper nutrition can also be a very valuable asset in helping to cope with the pressures of life. While there is no magic food or vitamin which automatically makes us peaceful and benign under the most intense pressures, there are foods which help us and foods which hurt us in coping with daily pressures. The foods that hurt us are the "junk foods" of various kinds, primarily because they fail to provide us with the nutrients necessary for proper physical and neurological health, and secondarily because they actually rob our bodies of certain valuable nutrients provided by more wholesome foods.

The wholesome foods which help our bodies include the protein-rich foods (primarily meat and dairy products), the whole grains (as well as seeds and nuts), the vegetables, and the fruits. Some people find that vitamin C, or a well-formulated B-complex vitamin supplement, or even brewer's yeast or food yeast (*not* baker's yeast) help them to cope better with daily stresses. (The B vitamins should always be taken in a well-balanced group—never singly unless prescribed by a physician.)

The stress-combating benefits of good nutrition are of both short-range and long-range value. Some people experience significantly improved stress-coping ability within a few days of instituting a proper, well-balanced diet, but almost everyone experiences this kind of effect after several weeks of careful eating, especially when accompanied by a sensible exercise program.

Moving and Meditating

One very obvious means of coping with excess stresses is to simply move away from them. Unfortunately, many people who relocate in order to get away from overwhelming problems finds themselves embroiled in a new set of problems which are just as overwhelming as the previous ones! However, there are cases where the pressures of urban living are so truly overwhelming that relocation to a more peaceful setting does indeed provide legitimate and effective relief. This whole issue of moving to escape from local problems is an extremely sensitive one that needs to be handled with careful thinking and a prayerful sensitivity to the will of God for the particular issue in question.

A recently popularized and still somewhat controversial technique for reducing personal feelings of tension is that of meditation and biofeedback. Dr. Herbert Benson of Boston has done experimental work in various behavioral techniques which help to relieve stress-induced disorders, particularly high blood pressure. He found that through a mental-concentration technique called biofeedback, many people are actually able to reduce their own blood pressure somewhat when properly trained to block out all their usual thoughts, concentrating instead on a single word or phrase. While Dr. Benson specifically included transcendental meditation in his experiments, he also acknowledges that other forms of meditation, not necessarily of Eastern origin, could have equal or even greater benefits.

For a born-again Christian, meditating on the written promises of God should certainly prove more beneficial and more tension-relieving than merely thinking pleasant thoughts or chanting a mantra. When God tells us, "I will never leave you nor forsake you," that is a promise worth appropriating for our own personal daily lives. The Apostle Paul, who certainly had more than his fair share of stresses in life, could recommend on the basis of his own personal experience, "Do not be anxious for anything, but in everything by prayer and supplication with thanksgiving let your requests be made known to God" (Philippians 4:6). Implicit trust in God is certainly the only *ultimate* answer to the pressures and tensions of our daily lives.

6 BODY IN MOTION

♦──────────────────────────────────────

Howard has been in the hospital for two full days now, and he has been told by Dr. Maynard, his attending physician, that he has experienced a myocardial infarction—a rather typical kind of heart attack which in Howard's case involved significant damage to the lower part of his heart.

Howard's earlier pain, nausea, weakness, and sense of impending doom had subsided considerably, but now he began to feel deeply depressed because of his uncertain future. "Will I ever be able to work again? How will I take care of my family? Will I ever be able to resume normal relations with my wife again?" As these thoughts went through Howard's mind, he experienced a significant loss of self-esteem; he was simply not a whole man anymore.

However, Dr. Maynard, a bright young specialist in internal medicine, assured Howard that with proper treatment he could be back to work in about two months, and that his life had the potential of becoming fully normal again. Howard's wife, Lois, echoed these same encouragements to him, and so did the pastor from the church of which Howard had nominally been a member. As a matter of fact, after one of the pastor's visits, Howard decided to make a major recommitment of his life to Christ.

Man Alive

During the next few days, all kinds of encouraging things seemed to happen. Howard was transferred out of the coronary care unit of the hospital and into a regular recuperation room, where he was able to sit up in a chair and even walk to the bathroom unassisted. Dr. Maynard told Howard that his heart was no longer skipping beats, that his pulse-rate was back to normal, that the damage to his heart had not been massive, and that his heart was still functioning reasonably well as a pump.

Howard felt slightly dizzy the first few times he got up from his chair, but otherwise he felt reasonably well. In fact, during his fourth day in the hospital, Howard felt so good that he told everyone, including Dr. Maynard, that he thought he was ready to leave the hospital and go home. However, Dr. Maynard informed Howard that his heart damage would not be rectified that quickly, and that he would need to remain hospitalized for the next week or two.

The next day the rehabilitation therapist showed Howard how to do certain simple exercises with his arms and supervised a regularly scheduled walking program. By now Howard felt surprisingly good. He was able to walk capably in the hallways of the hospital with no excessive rise in his pulse-rate. Howard felt more normal every day, and everyone was encouraged with his progress.

During Howard's third week in the hospital, Dr. Maynard told Howard he was ready to go home, and his family and friends were delighted. Howard was told that he would have to stay home for a couple of weeks, until his first appointment with Dr. Maynard, but that he would be able to walk around the house and do some light hobby work.

Howard in Motion

Two weeks later, Howard kept his appointment with Dr. Maynard and found that he was well enough to be placed on a moderate walking program. In another two weeks he visited Dr. Maynard again, and this time he was placed on a walking program which included longer and longer jaunts. At first these were only two or three blocks, but by the time Howard visited Dr. Maynard again he was walking well over a mile every day without feeling overly tired.

Less than two months after his coronary, Howard was walking three miles every day and feeling quite good about it. At this point he went back to work on a half-day schedule for a two-week trial period. Howard tolerated the work reasonably well, although he had to admit that he was glad to get home after each half-day's work, since he did tire more easily than before his heart attack. However, within a few weeks Howard was able to work a normal, full-day schedule without feeling overly tired.

Howard had heard of men who took up jogging after experiencing a heart attack, and so he talked to Dr. Maynard about this idea. Dr. Maynard responded by telling Howard that if he could pass a treadmill stress test, he might be able to begin jogging. Howard took the treadmill test, and even Dr. Maynard was surprised at how well he performed. Howard was told that he could immediately begin a supervised program of vigorous exercise. He was fortunate to find an opening in a cardiac rehabilitation program at his local YMCA. Howard bought himself a pair of jogging shoes and some shorts, and was delighted to begin his program of alternating walking and jogging.

Howard participated in this program faithfully three times a week for ten weeks, and by the end of the ten weeks he was able to jog continuously at a slow pace for nearly two miles without exceeding his maximum allowable pulse-rate. By the time Howard graduated from this supervised ten-week program, he felt better than he had in years, and he eagerly looked forward to his jogging, which he was soon enjoying nearly every day.

A year later Howard was still jogging—in fact, six miles every day—and he had never felt better in his life. He was now down to 165 pounds, his high school weight. His business affairs seemed to be going better than in previous years, and all of Howard's friends remarked about his exceptional energy and productivity. Even Dr. Maynard was surprised to find that Howard's serum-cholesterol level, which had once been 260 milligram percent, was now reduced to 180 through Howard's jogging program, sensible eating, and weight loss. His HDL level, which had once been a below-optimal 40, was now up to an excellent 60. His ratio of cholesterol to HDL, which had once been 6.5 (average male = 5.0), was down to a superb 3.0.

The events of the preceding year had been truly remarkable ones for Howard, for after suffering a frightening and depressing heart attack, he was now at the point where his likelihood of suffering another attack was probably less than that of the average male of his age!

How to Get Moving

If you are a typical American over 35 years of age, and if you are honest with yourself, you'll have to admit that you are somewhat like Howard was in the days before his heart attack. If you're a woman, remember that your comparative immunity to heart attacks begins to decrease rapidly once you pass menopause.

In the previous chapters we discussed various ways of coping with some of the most important heart-disease risk factors, and in this chapter we will be discussing the clinical importance of adequate exercise. The real secret of successful exercising is to find some form of health-building exercise that you can learn to truly enjoy. Brisk walking, running, bicycling, swimming, and cross-country skiing are all healthful forms of exercise, and many people find that they can sincerely enjoy one or more of these activities several times throughout every week of the year. For people who cannot exercise outdoors because of bad weather or other reasons, indoor jump-roping or stationary bicycling have often proven extremely satisfying, especially when done to the accompaniment of music or even certain kinds of TV.

The purpose of this chapter is to introduce you to the joys of adequate exercise and to provide you with enough basic information to help you get started soon and safely on an exercise program that will enrich your whole body for the rest of your life. (If you would like still more information about exercising after finishing this chapter, read the excellent booklet *Exercise Your Way to Fitness and Heart Health,* by Lenore R. Zohman, M.D., or the full-length book *The New Aerobics,* by Kenneth Cooper, M.D.)

Aerobic Exercise

We showed earlier in this book how a lack of regularly practiced vigorous exercise may be a major contributing factor to heart disease, and how regular vigorous exercise gives every promise of providing significant protection against the onset of coronary heart disease. We have reviewed some of the physiologic benefits of vigorous exercise, showing that improved heart, blood-vessel, and muscle function occur as a result of regular aerobic exercise. When practiced regularly, jogging or other forms of aerobic exercise have helped foster general good health, weight loss, and significant mental benefits, including reduced nervous tension, lifting of depression, clarified thinking, and even euphoric mood-uplifting.

We have said that *aerobic* exercise is the one kind of vigorous exercise which is truly effective in providing the above-mentioned benefits, and now we would like to define the term "aerobic." Aerobic exercise may be defined as any exercise which results in increased air or oxygen uptake by the body as a result of physically exercising the larger muscles of the body for a prolonged period of time. To be truly aerobic, the exercise must involve the larger skeletal muscles of the body and must be brisk enough so that the heart-rate or pulse-rate is increased significantly and the person is breathing somewhat more deeply and rapidly than normal, though not to the point of extreme breathlessness (resulting in oxygen debt, as in anaerobic exercise). Aerobic exercise, though vigorous, is steady and rhythmic, not punctuated by sudden outbursts of activity.

Nonaerobic Exercise

Many popular exercises which are commonly thought to be healthful are actually not aerobic at all and therefore do not provide the previously mentioned benefits in protecting against heart disease. In fact, some of these nonaerobic exercises may actually be dangerous to people with undiagnosed heart disease.

For example, isometric exercises involve minimal muscular movements with maximal muscular stress, often exercised against special motion-impeding isometric equipment. Because the muscles are working against an immovable or nearly immovable resistance, there is a temporary increase in blood pressure and a diminished flow of blood. Even weight-lifting, though it is not purely isometric, falls into this general category of high-resistance, minimum-motion exercise.

This is not to say that all such exercises are totally worthless; when done by healthy people free of heart disease (especially younger athletes), weight-lifting and other isometric-type exercises can be of some value in strengthening specific muscles (sometimes injured muscles) or even as part of a program of overall fitness to prevent injury. These benefits are especially obtainable when the heaviest weights or resistances are avoided. However, even when practiced under ideal conditions, isometric exercises do not provide any particular benefits to the cardiovascular system. In fact, it has actually been demonstrated that certain world-class weight-lifters when tested on a treadmill have actually had less aerobic capacity than the average unexercised individual!

Even such beneficial exercises as basketball, singles tennis, squash, handball, etc. (which are all largely aerobic) contain a certain element of danger, since they require occasional sudden bursts of high-energy output with accompanying high heartrates and high oxygen debt with its anaerobic accumulation of lactic acid, as well as other disadvantages. Any of these sports hold potential danger for people with un-diagnosed heart disease.

Snow shoveling has had an especially sinister rep-utation of being a widow-maker because it is often done against high resistance (heavy snow), rapidly to the point of being anaerobic (oxygen debt), and in adverse environmental conditions (cold winds). However, when done under the right conditions and at the proper pace, even snow-shoveling can be done aerobically and can be a comparatively safe exercise for most people.

Actually, even walking or jogging can be done at such a pace that they fall below or above the range of acceptable and safe aerobic exercise. For most people, slow-to-moderate walking is not a strenuous enough exercise to be truly aerobic, and for athletes in top condition even slow jogging may be too restful to be truly aerobic. On the other hand, for some people even slow jogging on level surfaces may be so strenuous that safe limits are exceeded and the exer-cise passes the point of being aerobic. (This is espe-cially true for jogging beginners.)

The Target Zone

These extreme situations illustrate the fact that there is a certain safe and optimal target zone of exercise. A number of studies have shown that such a target zone which is both safe and aerobic occurs within the range of 60 to 80 percent of a person's maximum aerobic power. This maximum aerobic power occurs at that point of maximal exercise when the heart and circulatory system cannot deliver any more oxygen to the body's tissues, and the exercise cannot be continued any longer or harder without approaching exhaustion. At this point not enough oxygen can be delivered for the muscles to continue working aerobically, and almost simultaneously the heart is unable to beat any faster.

For most normal, active individuals, the point of maximum aerobic power and maximum attainable heartrate are nearly identical, and the target zone of 60 to 80 percent of maximum aerobic power is about the same as the desirable 70 to 85 percent of maximum attainable heartrate. A person's maximum attainable heartrate can be determined quite accurately by physical testing on a treadmill or bicycle ergometer. However, statistical tables have been prepared which can predict with reasonable accuracy the maximim attainable heartrate of an average person, depending on his or her age. (One's maximum attainable heartrate decreases progressively with age.)

But even if a person lacks access to such tables, he can predict his approximate maximum heartrate by the

THE TARGET ZONE FOR AEROBIC EXERCISE

AGE IN YEARS	APPROXIMATE MINIMUM AEROBIC HEARTRATE (70% of Maximum Achievable)	APPROXIMATE MAXIMUM AEROBIC HEARTRATE (85% of Maximum Achievable)	APPROXIMATE MAXIMUM ACHIEVABLE HEARTRATE* (Roughly 220 Minus Age)
25	140	170	200
30	136	165	194
35	132	160	188
40	127	155	182
45	123	150	176
50	120	145	171
55	116	140	165
60	111	135	159
65	107	130	153

TARGET ZONE
(Desirable Range)

*Actual maximum heartrates vary somewhat among individuals, and some data show average maximum heartrates which vary somewhat from this table.

simple formula of 220 minus one's age in years. In other words, a 40-year-old man or woman would have an approximate maximum attainable heartrate of 220 minus 40, or 180, and a 60-year-old-man or woman would have an approximate maximum attainable heartrate of 220 minus 60, or 160.

Take Your Choice

This simple "target zone" principle shows that there are many exercises or chores that can be done aerobically by performing them at such a pace that the heartrate falls within the range of 70 to 85 percent of predicted maximum. Some of the most popular aerobic exercises include brisk walking, jogging, indoor or outdoor bicycling, swimming, rope jumping, running in place, aerobic dancing, and cross-country skiing. However, when done at the proper rate and for the proper length of time, even such chores as snow shoveling, lawn mowing (with a hand mower), and floor scrubbing can be done aerobically.

Dr. Lenore Zohman has recommended a five-to-ten minute period of warmup, stretching, or low-level exertion at about 50 percent of maximum heartrate, followed by 20 to 30 minutes of actual aerobic exercise in the target zone of 70 to 85 percent of maximum heartrate, followed by a five-to-ten-minute period of cool-down with gradually diminishing exercise. Such a composite of aerobic exercises should be performed three or preferably four times weekly.

Dr. Kenneth Cooper, author of *The New Aerobics* and *The Aerobics Way*, has approached the aerobics challenge by devising a point-scale system for many different kinds of commonly accepted aerobic exercises. His system involves attaining a weekly total of a certain number of aerobic exercise points (for example, 30 points a week), and this may involve varying amounts of time, depending on the kinds of exercise performed. Vigorous jogging, for example, would require less than one hour per week, while brisk walking could require as much as five hours per week or even more.

Dr. Ralph Paffenbarger's recent study of Harvard alumni (mentioned earlier in this book) demonstrated the protective effect against heart disease produced by 2000 kilocalories weekly of brisk exercise. Two thousand kilocalories of exercise weekly may be accomplished by any of the following:

1) walking 4 miles per hour 5 or 6 hours weekly;
2) playing singles tennis (not doubles) 45 to 60 minutes 5 times weekly (or some other schedule that results in 4 to 5 hours weekly);
3) bicycling 45 to 60 minutes at an average speed of 11 miles per hour 5 times weekly, or 12 miles per hour 4 times weekly, or some other combination resulting in 3 to 5 hours of bicycling weekly;

4) jogging 5.5 miles per hour for one hour 3 to 4 times weekly, or 6 miles per hour for one hour 3 times weekly, or some other combination totaling 3 hours weekly;

5) playing squash or handball one hour 3 times weekly.

No Reckless Plunge

Before actually beginning any aerobic exercise program, be sure to take stock of your overall physical condition. I recommend a complete physical checkup as part of an overall evaluation of your health and as the proper means of discovering any previously undiagnosed problems that might interfere with a vigorous exercise program, such as diabetes, hypertension, anemia, and especially heart disease.

Before beginning any vigorous new exercise program, anyone who has significant or multiple heart-disease risk factors (heredity, smoking, obesity, high blood fats, high blood pressure, etc.) or is above 35 to 40 years of age (particularly males) should probably be tested with either a bicycle ergometer or a treadmill stress test.* Any problems that are uncovered should be treated adequately (for example, bringing blood pressure down to a safe level), so that the aerobic exercise program can be started safely.

---

*Neither of these tests is a flawlessly accurate indicator of heart health, especially among relatively healthy younger people.

It is not wise to eat heavily shortly before vigorous exercise; either eat more lightly or wait two hours after a heavy meal. If you have a chest cold, flu, or other systemic infection, you should consider suspending your exercise program until these symptoms improve. If you exercise outdoors, you should try to avoid the most extreme weather conditions (cold, heat, precipitation, wind, etc.) or at least take proper steps to combat the extreme conditions. With proper timing and well-chosen clothing, most people can continue a healthful aerobic exercise program almost year-round.

Walk Before You Run?

For most people, the best beginning exercise is walking, since walking can be done by people of almost all ages and is the most natural exercise for the body, even more natural than jogging. To begin a walking program, first check your resting pulse-rate by putting the fingertips of your right hand to the left side of your neck (vice versa if you are left-handed) and checking the pulse of the main ("carotid") artery. Or you can place the fingertips of your right hand on the wrist of your left hand near the base of the thumb (vice versa if you are left-handed), although this pulse may be harder to feel than the neck pulse during or immediately after vigorous exercise.

With a little experimenting, you will be able to find your pulse quickly in one of these two locations.

Because the pulse-rate of most people drops quickly as soon as exercise is stopped, the best way to determine the number of heartbeats per minute is to count the number of beats in ten seconds and multiply this number by six.

Start your walking program on level or nearly level surfaces if possible, and after the first few minutes of walking take your pulse for ten seconds (stopping walking if necessary) and multiply by six. Have you reached your target zone of 70 to 85 percent of maximum predicted heartrate? If you are 40 years old, this is between 126 and 153 beats per minute, and if you are 50 years old it is between 112 and 135 beats per minute. If you have not reached your target rate, walk a little more briskly; if you have exceeded it, slow down a little.

A simple exertion test that applies to both walking and running is the "talk test." If you are walking or running at a proper aerobic pace, you should be exercising briskly but should still be able to speak comfortably with a partner, without experiencing undue breathlessness. If you are not in good physical condition, you might not be able to walk much more than half a mile, but if you are in fairly good condition, you might be able to walk a desirable three or four miles on your first day.

If you are overweight, arthritic, or just plain out of condition, be conservative and start with only about a half-mile of walking a day, but do it daily (or nearly every day) that first week. During the second week walk three-quarters of a mile each day, the third week one mile each day, etc., adding a quarter-mile per day per week until you eventually reach a desirable total of three or four miles daily. You muscles and joints may complain somewhat at first, and you may feel a little breathless, but if you start out moderately and continue consistently, you will be surprised at the gratifying progress that you make within just a few weeks.

Walking may take more time than jogging or other vigorous exercises to achieve and maintain aerobic fitness, but it is a safe form of exercise with little chance of injury, and to many people it is highly relaxing. Some middle-aged people and most elderly people should probably never progress beyond consistent aerobic walking.

Ready for Running?

If you are in reasonably good condition, and especially if you are already walking or undertaking some other gentle aerobic exercise program, or if you are a very busy person who would like to achieve and maintain aerobic fitness with a minimum expenditure of time, or even if you just like the thought of running, then consider the challenge of jogging.

Although jogging is an exceptionally fine form of aerobic exercise, it does have its drawbacks, especially for nonathletic, sedentary, or older persons. Joggers may develop foot injuries, tendon problems, shin splints, and abnormalities of the knees, hips, or back. In many cases these problems can be prevented or corrected by wearing proper shoes, by doing stretching exercises, by doing strengthening exercises for the abdomen, and in some cases by wearing special shoe inserts (called ''orthotics'') prescribed by a qualified podiatrist. Some people seem to get along fine with almost any kind of comfortable shoe, but for many people jogging shoes are so much more comfortable than conventional shoes, and they so greatly reduce the number of injuries, that they make the difference between continuing a jogging program or giving up in discouragement.

Do not begin a jogging program until you have shown that you are able to maintain a consistent aerobic walking program of from 15 to 24 miles weekly. You could then choose a jogging route of about one or two miles in length, and then alternately walk and jog that entire distance, jogging perhaps 50 yards or until your pulse-rate moves into the proper zone (or until you are just a little breathless) and then walking another 50 yards or paces. Continue alternating this way unless your legs are beginning to feel the strain of the newly begun jogging, and then walk the remainder of the distance. If your legs are quite sore the next day, do only walking during that day. Even if your legs feel quite good, it might be wise to do mostly walking on the second day of your walking-jogging program.

During the first whole week of your new program you could alternate walking-only days with walking-jogging days. After the first week, you could try more jogging and less walking, gradually moving into jogging only on alternate days or even every day. It may take several weeks to reach the point of mostly jogging, especially for out-of-condition, overweight, or older people, but most well-motivated people who are not seriously overweight can eventually reach the point where they are able to jog continuously several miles every other day.

The Joys of Jogging

Lest you think you would never be able to jog several miles continuously, Dr. Jack Scaff, a cardiologist from Hawaii, has claimed that almost anyone can learn to run a 26-mile marathon if he builds up jogging distances gradually over a period of about nine months. Dr. Scaff has had remarkable jogging success even with many of his patients who had already experienced a heart attack and with other patients whose coronary arteries were so severely narrowed that they could not even sustain a bypass operation.

I have been personally thrilled to participate with two most interesting groups of men in the world-famous Boston Marathon: one group came with Dr. Scaff of Hawaii, and the other group came with Dr. Terence Kavanagh of Toronto, and both groups consisted of formerly defeated and depressed heart-attack victims who were now in fine enough physical condition to run the entire 26 miles of this grueling event! (See Dr. Kavanagh's excellent book entitled *Heart Attack: Counterattack.*)

While it is not realistic to claim that everyone should or could become a marathon runner, a rapidly-increasing number of peple are learning to enjoy the exhilaration of jogging for fun and health. Jogging should be enjoyed; a daily or alternate-day jogging program should not be undertaken as a series of record-breaking races, with maximal or near-maximal exertion, since this kind of effort may actually result in increased stress, fatigue, and failure to relax. For most people, the greatest benefit of jogging comes not from a grueling, breathless pace, but from a medium aerobic pace in which a conversation could be carried on while running.

For some people, especially younger athletes in excellent condition, a hard-driving pace or even a racing pace provides a special competitive thrill, whether racing alone against the clock or racing against other runners; however, the typical American would be well-advised to begin his or her jogging program under the moderate conditions described in the preceding paragraph.

A realistic and desirable goal for most joggers is to patiently and persistently build up their jogging ability over a period of many months so that they can eventually enjoy the thrill of running effortlessly over hill and dale, through field and forest, along sandy beaches and even rocky trails.

There is a definite exhilaration, a euphoria, that most runners experience when they have developed to the point where they can easily cover several miles at a time without straining in the least. At that point it is possible to enjoy the sights and sounds of nature with a special delight. There is often a sense of freedom, of mastery, of expansiveness when one can cover distances and go to places that were once unthinkably difficult.

The Jolts of Jogging

Unfortunately, even jogging has its drawbacks. Sometimes jogging tends to produce injuries in certain muscles and joints (as mentioned previously), and jogging can also produce an imbalance in development of certain muscles. For example, the propelling muscles (calves, hamstrings, and lower back) can become somewhat overdeveloped as compared to the opposing muscles (shin muscles, thigh quadricep muscles, and abdominal muscles). This partial imbalance can be largely overcome by exercising the underdeveloped muscles with certain kinds of activity, such as bent-leg sit-ups for the abdomen muscles, stair-climbing and bicycling for the quadricep thigh muscles, and brisk walking for the shin muscles (and sometimes also for the quadricep

107

thigh muscles). Other special exercises can also be used to help joggers maintain total balance in their muscular development.

Sometimes the propelling muscles (those of the calves, hamstrings, and lower back) become somewhat shortened through jogging and should be stretched frequently through regular exercises, preferably done just before and after jogging. A simple stretching exercise for the hamstrings and back could include simply sitting on the floor with straightened legs before you, then gradually and steadily reaching for your toes, thereby putting a persistent stretch on these muscles for several seconds at a time. Calf muscles may be effectively stretched by standing in bare feet or stockinged feet two or three feet away from a wall and then leaning toward the wall. Numerous other special exercises have also been devised in order to help stretch the muscles of the legs and other parts of the body.

Many excellent books on running are now available, and one of the best of these is *The Complete Book of Running,* by James Fixx (published by Random House).

Cars, Canines, and Criminals

Sometimes both walkers and joggers have to face dangerous road traffic, especially in the cities and suburbs, and this can present a real safety problem. However, with some searching most walkers and joggers are able to find a safe place to exercise, even if it means driving a few miles to get there. If forced to use roads without sidewalks, walk or jog against the oncoming traffic, as far to the left as possible. Nighttime walking or jogging on such roads should be avoided if at all possible, but if this is not possible, then be sure to wear light-colored or reflective clothing.

Dogs can sometimes be a problem (and occasionally even other kinds of animals), and when possible dogs should not be directly challenged, especially when they are guarding their own turf or are with their masters. Dogs that chase you can sometimes be frightened away by turning quickly toward them and maintaining an aggressive stance. If a dog gets too aggressive, he can usually be quickly dispensed by rapping him briskly over the snout with a strong stick carried for this purpose.

In some areas, any walker or jogger, and especially a woman, will have to be on guard for molesters. The danger can be reduced by walking or jogging in the morning hours or by using some safe neighborhood within reasonable driving distance, by walking or jogging with a friend or group of friends, or by jogging with a large dog.

The Wheels Are Turning

Bicycling has also become a very popular exercise, since with the proper equipment it can be done either outdoors or indoors. On level terrain, almost any bicycle in safe condition can prove satisfactory, but in hilly country, three-, five-, or ten-speed bicycles make cycling much more enjoyable. Bicycling requires special precautions in road traffic and on rough, sandy, or slippery surfaces, as on ice and snow. Bicycling requires traveling about three or four times as far as jogging in order to produce the same aerobic benefit, but one advantage to this necessary extra distance is that it sometimes affords a greater variety of interesting scenery.

One advantage of bicycling over jogging is that bicycling involves much less risk of injury to joints and muscles. However, bicycling favors development of the antigravity muscles, especially quadriceps and calves, rather than a perfectly balanced development. "Saddle-soreness" can usually be alleviated by using a properly designed seat, although a few days or weeks may be required for the soreness to completely disappear. Overall, the aerobic benefits of bicycling and jogging are about equal if each is undertaken properly.

Indoor cycling on a stationary bicycle has important advantages, including accessibility in all seasons and in all kinds of weather. A well-made indoor exercising cycle may cost between 100 and 400 dollars, but after this initial outlay it involves virtually no further expense. Indoor cycling can be somewhat boring, but the exercise can be made much more interesting by the accompaniment of music, TV watching, or even reading. Many people schedule their indoor cycling to coincide with a favorite half-hour TV program, thereby killing two birds with one stone and at the same time having a daily reminder to do their exercise.

Indoor stationary cycling is especially therapeutic for people with cardiovascular diseases, including both angina pectoris with chest pressure as well as intermittent claudication with leg cramps that occur when exercising. When discomfort occurs, people with these problems simply stop cycling and remain seated until the discomfort goes away, either through temporary rest or with the additional help of nitroglycerin. Then they simply resume their therapeutic cycling.

The indoor stationary cycle is especially suitable for older people and those with problems of balance, one-sided weakness, prior stroke, etc., since there is no great difficulty in maintaining balance and very little danger of sudden falls. I have seen indoor cycling help produce a number of near-miraculous improvements in former invalids who had had marked coronary heart disease, angina pectoris, poor leg circulation, and even neurological problems. Most elderly people are able either to walk or to use an indoor cycle, thus helping to rejuvenate themselves with either of these two forms of excellent exercise.

Jogging and Jumping

There are two other popular forms of indoor aerobic exercise that can easily be done at home and have been particularly appealing to women.

Jogging in place can be done on a cushioned mat or rug and provides almost the same aerobic benefit as outdoor jogging, assuming that the optimum heart-rate has been achieved and maintained for the proper length of time.

A somewhat more difficult indoor exercise is "jump-roping" or "rope-skipping." The way this exercise is usually done results in rapid onset of very high heartrates, and therefore tends to be a very hard exercise for a beginner. However, if a rope-skipping program can be started slowly enough, with enough short interruptions to keep the heartrate within the proper range, and if each session of rope-skipping can be continued for a desirable 20 minutes or more, then this form of indoor exercise can develop physical endurance and can become a desirable form of aerobic exercise.

Both rope-skipping and jogging in place are especially appealing to younger women, since they can remain indoors, watch their children, and remain out of the eyesight of neighbors, friends, and other prying eyes. Many women have been good at rope-skipping in childhood and find that they can get back to it fairly easily. However, rope-skipping is probably too difficult for most elderly men and women.

Wonders in the Water?

Swimming is also an excellent form of exercise which provides great aerobic benefit. Swimming involves more muscles of the body than almost any other kind of exercise, although the greatest expenditure of effort is in the muscles of the arms and upper torso. (The legs are exercised relatively little and do not add much to propulsion. The antigravity muscles are hardly exercised at all.) Swimming in suitable pools or other areas also involves the problem of financial expense, lack of universal availability, and often crowding. Also, swimming tends to be a seasonal form of exercise for many people, and considerable time and distance are often involved in getting to the swimming area. Many people are unable to swim efficiently, and some cannot swim at all.

Nevertheless, swimming can be an excellent form of exercise, especially for people with injured muscles, ligaments, and joints of the legs. Swimming is a smooth, rhythmic exercise that involves no jerking and less resistance than most land exercises. The buoyancy of the water helps to support the body, further aiding people with injuries and allowing them to get the arerobic exercise that everybody needs. Injured athletes often recover remarkably while undergoing a program of swimming. For many people who are permanently crippled, swimming has become an excellent, lifelong form of enjoyable aerobic exercise.

The Special Joys of Winter

An especially excellent form of aerobic exercise is cross-country skiing (ski-touring). This involves the use of narrow, light skis which are not fixed at the heel (to allow for a rhythmic, walking-gliding action). About one-third of the propelling force comes from the use of the poles and two-thirds from the legs, making this aerobic exercise one of the best-balanced in the proportionate use of the arm and leg muscles. In cross-country skiing there is less strain on the joints than in jogging, although there is some risk of injury due to falls (but much less risk than in downhill skiing).

In addition to being an exceptionally fine form of aerobic exercise, cross-country skiing offers outstanding aesthetic appeal in pristine wilderness settings. For these reasons and others, this kind of skiing is rapidly becoming one of the most popular forms of aerobic exercise.

Do It Yourself

Our brief survey has suggested that there are a whole multitude of exercises that can be performed aerobically, and the list is not confined to the specific examples that we have given. Almost everyone should be able to find some form of aerobic exercise that is both practical and appealing for his or her circumstances. With a little imagination you can even devise your own form of aerobic exercise. Wood-cutting, canoe-paddling, lawn-mowing, scrubbing and sweeping floors, and many other activities can be done aerobically if the heartrate is brought up to the optimum range and kept there for an adequate period of time.

I have had one elderly female patient who does daily aerobic walking in a long hallway of her apartment. Another patient, an elderly man, has a large basement in which he walks back and forth briskly to meet his aerobic requirement. A third patient, an elderly man who previously had experienced a heart attack, does his aerobic walking daily in a large indoor shopping mall, thereby avoiding extremes of cold, snow, heat, or humidity.

The most important thing is to find some form of suitable aerobic exercise that you can enjoy, and then stick to it regularly so that your weekly aerobic requirements are met. By doing this you become eligible for the benefits of a more efficient heart and circulatory system, an overall improved sense of well-being, a greater clarity of thinking, an enhanced relaxation and mood-uplifting, and the increased opportunity to enjoy a healthy heart. Adequate aerobic exercise may add years to your life and will certainly add life to your years!

7 EAT FOR YOUR LIFE

Very likely you have heard the popular saying, "You are what you eat," and there is much truth in this statement. Our bodily development and the continuing maintenance of the health of all body tissues depends in large part on the foods and beverages we consume.

In much of the world, especially in the so-called "third world" or underdeveloped countries, food deprivation or even starvation because of a lack of even the most basic food requirements is a major problem. However, in the United States and most of the developed Western nations, the major nutritional problem is that of overconsumption of high-calorie foods with its accompanying phenomenon of obesity. Estimates based on reliable surveys indicate that as many as 80 million Americans may be overweight, with 30 million at least 20 percent overweight and 15 million seriously overweight.

In addition to the problem of overweight caused by overconsumption of high-calorie foods, many Americans also suffer from insufficient intake of certain vital food elements. In this chapter we will survey the basic elements of good nutrition in order to help you combat overweight, achieve and maintain vibrant general health, and increase your resistance to such scourges as heart disease and cancer. We will begin by reviewing the seven basic nutritional constituents required by the human body.

Water

Because the human body consists of about 50 to 70 percent water, sufficient daily intake of water or water-containing fluids is essential to life itself for every single individual. No one can reach or maintain optimum health without sufficient daily intake of water in the form of food, beverages, and/or plain water itself. A useful rule of thumb for daily water intake is to drink enough water so that at least once during every 24-hour period the urine becomes water-diluted to the point that it is relatively clear and colorless.

The presence of pollutants in public water supplies is becoming an increasing problem in the U.S., and one which we should combat by any practical means possible. If the purity of your public water supply is not what it should be, you might try pure spring or well water from a reliable source, or even a home water purifier or distiller.

Public water supplies can contain low-to-moderate levels of various kinds of substances which are foreign to the human body, but usually the single greatest pollutant is chlorine, which is added to many public water supplies in order to inhibit the growth of harmful microorganisms. While water chlorination is remarkably successful in protecting people againt infectious diseases, there is some evidence that it may have certain harmful effects on the human body, especially when combined with certain kinds of organic materials. There is even a possibility that water chlorination may have a slight cancer-producing effect.

Artificially softened water (not to be confused with purified or distilled water) should never be used for human consumption because it often contains excess sodium (the salt that may aggravate high blood pressure or heart disease), as well as other unwanted elements, such as lead. Aside from the presence of chlorine or various pollutants, hard water is a healthful beverage because the calcium and magnesium which make water "hard" may serve as a partial protection against heart disease. (Present evidence suggests that silicon in water may also provide some protection.) High-quality spring waters are usually hard waters which are free of harmful pollutants.

Proteins

The amino acids which make up proteins are the building blocks of our bodies from which all muscles, bones, organs, tissues, and blood are constructed.

The human body can manufacture certain amino acids from certain other amino acids, but there are a select few "essential" amino acids which must be present in the digestive system simultaneously (in other words, eaten at almost the same time) in order for any useful growth, construction, or repair of the body to occur.

Good sources of high-quality protein which contain all the essential amino acids include the following: meats, fish, eggs, milk, and soybeans. It is highly desirable to eat at least some complete protein (containing all the essential amino acids) at every meal. A useful rule of thumb for daily protein intake is one gram of protein for every kilogram of body weight, or about 70 grams of protein daily for a 154-pound man. (Some nutritionists feel that only about half this amount is necessary, especially if the protein is of high quality.)

Fats

Certain essential fatty acids are required by the human body in order to maintain good health. Of the two basic kinds of fats, saturated and unsaturated, the more important kind for human health is unsaturated. In fact, overconsumption of saturated fats (a common problem in the United States) contributes to heart disease and elevated blood-cholesterol levels with subsequent atherosclerosis.

The animal fats are generally saturated and usually solid at room temperature, while the vegetable fats or oils are usually unsaturated (technically polyunsaturated) and are generally liquid at room temperature. For most people the best source of polyunsaturated fatty acids is one or two tablespoonsful daily of liquid vegetable oil which is polyunsaturated, perhaps used as a dressing on a salad or other raw food.

Americans currently consume about 42 percent of their daily caloric intake in fats, with 16 percent of total calories as saturated fats, and 26 percent as poly- and monounsaturated fats. In February 1977 the Select Committee on Nutrition and Human Needs of the United States Senate published the report "Dietary Goals for the United States," which recommended reducing calories from fat intake to only about 30 percent of the total (10 percent saturated and 20 percent poly- and monounsaturated).

Nathan Pritikin, of Southern California, has recommended an even more drastic reduction of fats, to only 10 percent of the total daily calories consumed, with the remainder of the diet to consist of 10 percent protein and 80 percent natural, unrefined carbohydrates ("complex carbohydrates"). He also recommends a daily cholesterol intake of only 5 milligram percent, as opposed to the usual 600 to 750 milligram percent. Hopefully, this low intake would not only prevent atherosclerosis (hardening of the arteries) from taking place, but would actually encourage reversal of existing atherosclerosis.

It is almost certainly safe to say that Americans

should consume considerably less animal fat, using polyunsaturated vegetable oils instead. A word of caution: all nonliquid oleomargines, even those made from corn oil, are at least partly saturated by a special hydrogen-adding process in order to prevent them from liquefying at room temperature.

In addition, the chemical configuration of these artificially saturated fats is different from that of natural saturated fats, and in some animal studies the artificially saturated fats have been shown to cause more atherosclerosis than natural fats such as butter.

Very recently, some scientists have expressed a concern that a dietary shift from saturated fats to polyunsaturated fats, while helpful in preventing cardiovascular disease, may increase susceptibility to certain kinds of cancer. However, I personally would continue to recommend using natural, fresh, polyunsaturated fats (oils) in reasonable amounts, while at the same time taking the extra precaution of using supplementary antioxidants, such as vitamins C and E.

Carbohydrates

Carbohydrates, including starches and sugars, are a legitimate and important source of calories, providing energy needed by our bodies to carry out all daily functions, incuding physical exercise. Many people seem to feel that all carbohydrates are harmful and should be eliminated from the diet, but this is a half-truth at best because the complex carbohydrates consist of natural starches and sugars as they come from foods (especially fruits, vegetables, and grains) and are very beneficial to the human body in this natural state. These complex carbohydrates, including most unprocessed cereal grains, breads, rice, vegetables, potatoes, etc., have been the mainstay in the diet of most of the world's peoples throughout history.

The great change that has occurred in the developed Western nations in this century has been the dramatically increased consumption of *refined* carbohydrates (especially white sugar or sucrose), which is being increasingly recognized as very harmful to human health. Americans today consume about 40 to 50 percent of their total calories in the form of carbohydrates, of which 22 percent consists of complex carbohydrates and 24 percent consists of sugar. Most Americans actually consume more low-quality calories from sugar than they do high-quality calories from the beneficial complex carbohydrates.

The Select Committee on Nutrition and Human Needs of the United States Senate has recommended consuming 58 percent of all calories as carbohydrates, with a large 40 to 45 percent as complex carbohydrates and only 15 percent as sugar. Nathan Pritikin has recommended consuming about 80 percent of all calories as carbohydrates, but consisting almost totally of complex carbohydrates rather than sugars (including sugar, honey, and molasses).

In their natural state, the complex carbohydrates

include not only the desirable slow-burning starches, but also an abundant supply of natural fibers, vitamins, and minerals, including the crucial trace elements. The refining of grain cereals, dominant since the turn of the century, has resulted in the removal of the germ and the bran of wheat, leaving a white-flour product which is then made into bread that now lacks much of the fiber, vitamins, trace minerals, and even proteins that are present in bread made from whole grains.

The dramatic increase since the turn of the century in the processing and consumption of highly refined sugar has resulted in a tremendous intake of "empty" calories—calories which contain no other nutritional elements and are devoid of any other nutritional benefits. This great American empty-calorie binge results in simultaneous overweight and undernourishment, because these sugary calories are eaten in place of truly nourishing foods and because the mere bodily metabolism of these sugary products uses up extra amounts of certain vitamins in the body, especially thiamine. In people who eat sugary snacks instead of nourishing food, the empty-calorie habit may lead to or aggravate diabetes or hypoglycemia. In many people, a sugary snack quickly produces a temporary higher-than-normal blood sugar level, followed by a lower-than-normal blood sugar level with accompanying exhaustion and depression.

Minerals

Minerals for human consumption are generally classified as macrominerals (including salts) and microminerals. Macrominerals are those minerals required by the human body in relatively large amounts: calcium, phosphorous, magnesium, potassium, sodium, fluorine, and the sulfur-containing compounds.

Calcium and phosphorous are particularly needed for the formation and maintenance of bones. Calcium is also critically necessary for the blood-clotting mechanism, and phosphorous plays a vital role in the controlled release of energy derived from carbohydrates, fats, and proteins. Magnesium is vital for intracellular metabolism, including proper function of the heart, and it is also required for the synthesis of protein. Sodium (as in sodium chloride, common table salt) and potassium serve as electroytes which help maintain proper fluid balances in the body.

The microminerals are those minerals which are vitally essential to the human body, but are required only in small amounts. These are sometimes called trace minerals, and they include iron, iodine, copper, zinc, manganese, cobalt, selenium, molybdenum, chromium, fluorine, vanadium, tin, nickel, and silicon. These microminerals are involved in a multitude of bodily functions, including enzyme function, oxygen utilization, cellular metabolism, etc. Both macrominerals and microminerals are pres-

THE JOY OF GOOD HEALTH

ent in adequate amounts in most natural, unrefined foods, but the microminerals especially are refined out of many modern foods by present-day processing methods.

Vitamins

There are two major kinds of vitamins: oil- or fat-soluble and water-soluble. The oil- or fat-soluble vitamins include A, D, E, and K. The water-soluble vitamins include C (ascorbic acid) and the B-complex vitamins: thiamine (B-1), riboflavin (B-2), niacin, pyridoxine (B-6), panthothenic acid, folic acid, cyanocobalamin (B-12), biotin, and choline. Recommended daily allowances have been established for most of the vitamins.

Surplus amounts of oil-soluble vitamins tend to be stored in the human body, and for this reason very high doses of Vitamins A, D, E, and K should not be taken for a prolonged period, since this can sometimes result in dangerous toxicity. However, adequate amounts of Vitamin A are necessary for proper bone growth, adequate nighttime vision, and the general health of the skin and body tissues. Vitamin A may also help strengthen the enamel layer of the teeth. Vitamin D is essential for proper metabolism of calcium and phosphorous, and for proper bone growth. Vitamin E is an antioxidant which may help to preserve other vitamins, to aid in oxygenation of body tissues, and possibly to protect against toxins and aging. Vitamin K is essential for proper blood-clotting.

The water-soluble vitamins (C and B-complex) are not stored to any great extent in the human body, and a fresh supply of them is therefore needed daily. Vitamin C aids in the construction of all body tissues, as it is sort of a cellular glue that helps hold together connective tissues, blood vessels, bones, etc. Vitamin C also helps protect the function of other vitamins and may also help protect against toxins and infections, and may even help promote longevity. The B vitamins are particularly involved in the release of energy from carbohydrates, fats, and proteins. They also help protect the body against toxins and infectious disease, they help the nervous system to function smoothly, and they aid in the synthesis and metabolism of proteins and in the formation of red blood cells.

As with the minerals, all of these vitamins are found in adequate amounts in fresh, wholesome, natural foods which have not been refined or destroyed by excessive cooking or other destructive processing. Many of the vitamins and trace minerals act as enzymes, helping bodily functions to take place smoothly.

Fiber and Bulk

Because food fiber contains no real nutritive value in and of itself, and because it is not absorbed by the body from the gastrointestinal tract, it was in past years considered of little value in human nutrition. In recent years, however, the beneficial effect of fiber and bulk has become more clearly realized; the proper functioning of the gastrointestinal tract, particularly the lower colon, is now known to depend partly on the presence of adequate food fiber and bulk.

British researchers, including Dr. Denis Burkitt, have described the adverse effects which native African blacks experienced when they gave up their normal fiber-rich diet in order to enjoy the refined white man's diet of the Western world. The once-healthy Africans eventually fell prey to such diseases of civilization as constipation, diverticulosis, diverticulitis, appendicitis, bowel cancer, hemorrhoids, varicose veins, gallbladder disease, hiatus hernia, and possibly diabetes mellitus and heart disease. Fruits, vegetables, and especially unrefined cereal grains contain all the fiber (bran) needed for normal functioning of the bowels and for helpful protection against the just-mentioned serious diseases. The importance of bran in the diet can hardly be overemphasized.

Choose Your Foods

While it is important to be aware of the health significance of the seven major nutritional constituents that we have just discussed, it is even more important to learn how to consume these constituents in proper, balanced amounts, Even though some of these constituents can be purchased as individual entities (liquid protein, individual vitamins and minerals, etc.), wholesome nutrition requires more than just the casual mixing of individual food components. In other words, good nutritional health requires well-chosen foods that are both appetizing and health-building.

These health-building requirements can be adequately met by choosing wisely from among the four major groups of wholesome foods, including:

> The proteins
> The fruits and vegetables
> The dairy products
> The cereals, grains, and breads.

Millions of children in America have been taught that these four major groups of food build good health, and sound research seems to indicate that this is indeed the case.

The Proteins

The protein group, consisting of meat, fish, eggs, and legumes (such as soybeans), are rich in protein and the essential amino acids needed by the body for growth and repair. (Despite their high protein content, some nutritionists classify the legumes under the "fruits and vegetables" category.)

True vegetarians (their number now increasing in this country) do not consume any meats, fish, or eggs, nor do they consume any milk or dairy products. However, most vegetarians today are lacto-ovo vegetarians, consuming both milk products and eggs along with foods from vegetable sources. (True vegetarians get their protein and essential amino acids only from a proper selection of various cereals, grains, and legumes.) Vegetarianism requires a good knowledge of nutrition in order to obtain sufficient daily protein, but it can be done, as shown in *Diet for a Small Planet,* by Frances Moore Lappe.

However, I feel that for most Americans it is still advisable to choose at least one item daily from the protein group in order to receive an adequate amount of high-quality protein. The idea is not to eliminate all meat and dairy proteins, but simply to choose the best of such proteins. Beef, pork, lamb, eggs, and whole-milk products are all high in saturated fats and cholesterol, and for this reason none of these foods should be eaten in great quantities. Also, these foods are rather expensive sources of protein because of the resources required to produce them. For example, it takes 7 to 20 pounds of grain to produce a single pound of edible beef!

Even though almost all meats provide ample amounts of certain vitamins and minerals (as well as proteins), certain meats have an especially favorable balance of nutrients. Fish, for example, is high in protein but low in saturated fats, and fish in general, especially saltwater fish, also contain many other necessary trace minerals.

Although high in cholesterol and saturated fats,

eggs contain protein of very high quality. Some people should restrict their consumption of eggs because of a problem with cholesterol and saturated fats, but if consumption of meat and dairy products decreases, then egg consumption can be increased somewhat. Legumes, especially soybeans, are often rich in high-quality protein (depending on the kind of legume), and the fat content is both low and polyunsaturated. A certain amount of complete protein (containing all essential amino acids) should be consumed at every meal.

The Fruits and Vegetables

The fruits and vegetables are rich in vitamins, minerals, fiber, and carbohydrates, but low in protein (except for legumes). If possible, some yellow and green vegetables, including some of the leafy variety, should be eaten every day, along with two servings of natural fruit (unsugared). The natural sugars contained in fruit are combined with many other beneficial nutritional factors, and are therefore highly preferred over refined sugar and even over such highly concentrated natural sweets as honey and molasses.

Potatoes are a good, wholesome food that has been much maligned in the recent past. Much like bread and cereal grains, potatoes were for many years a staff of life for such diverse societies as Andean Indians (one of the earliest cultivators of potatoes) and Europeans, especially the Irish. Potatoes are not as high in

131

calories as most people imagine (only about 75 to 100 calories per potato, roughly the same as a similarly sized apple). The real problem is that the number of calories in potatoes themselves is doubled or tripled by the addition of butter, cream, or sauces. Potatoes are rich in fiber, potassium, and other important minerals, and even Vitamin C. The starch in potatoes is a wholesome source of complex carbohydrates, and potatoes are even a fair source of protein.

The Dairy Products

The dairy products include milk, true cheeses (not artificial, nondairy cheeses), yogurt, and high-butter-fat-content products such as butter and real ice cream (not artificial, nondairy ice cream). Most Americans would be well-advised to reduce their consumption of butterfat found in ice cream, butter, fatty cheeses, and whole milk. All milk should not be eliminated, since it is a very complete food, especially for infants and growing children. Even for adults, milk provides valuable protein as well as calcium and other important minerals. Low-fat milk, buttermilk, and yogurt are valuable sources of reduced-fat protein. Since cheeses can vary widely in their fat and salt content, all available information on cheese labels needs to be read very carefully, especially by people who have heart disease, high blood fats, high blood pressure, or even excessive body weight.

A significant percentage of adults in America have

lost the intestinal enzyme that digests milk sugar. After drinking fresh milk (not buttermilk or other forms of soured milk),they may get a form of colitis with gas, diarrhea, abdominal cramps, and possibly other symptoms, all caused by the fermentation of milk sugar that takes place in their intestines. This problem can be completely eliminated by substituting some form of milk product that has already been soured, such as buttermilk, yogurt, or cheese. Many adults have little or no deficiency of the enzyme that digests milk sugar and can therefore continue to drink moderate amounts of fresh milk, perhaps a pint daily.

The Cereals, Grains, and Breads

As we mentioned previously, bread has been the staff of life for many people of the world for hundreds of years. However, the airy, light, bleached white loaves that we see lining our supermarket shelves today are so devitalized of the grains' original nutrients and so loaded with preservatives and various chemicals that they can in no way be compared with the staff of life that has developed strong people and nations in the past. Thankfully, today there is a resurgence of interest in real whole-grain bread that is wholesome to eat because it is nutritionally sound. Since the turn of the century, when grain began to be refined in large quantities, most of our breads have been largely deprived of a whole series of valuable nutrients which were either thrown away or fed to animals. When the bran and the germ of the wheat are removed, the resulting product not only deprives people of valuable protein, B-vitamins, and trace minerals, but it also eliminates the roughage or fiber represented by bran.

I recommend emphatically that only whole grains be consumed for optimum health—only whole-wheat bread, whole-grain cereals, and whole natural brown rice. For those people whose living situations require them to continue eating white bread and refined cereals, wheat germ and bran supplementation can be extremely helpful. The advertisers of white bread have made much of the fact that their products are supplemented with several vitamins, but what they fail to mention is that most of the B-vitamins are not included in the supplementation, and that trace minerals are usually also excluded.

Because even whole-grain breads, cereals, and other whole-grain products consist primarily of carbo-hydrates, many people fear that to eat such foods will lead to obesity. Certainly no one should overeat whole-grain products merely because they are nourishing foods, but the fear that eating whole-grain breads and cereals inevitably leads to overweight should be laid to rest by the fact that millions of peo-ple in the world today live largely on such breads and cereals, yet continue to remain lean and trim their en-tire lives. This is partly because wholesome breads, cereals, and grains with their associated bran are somewhat filling and tend to provide a feeling of fullness, thereby helping to prevent overeating. The average person who stays reasonably active physically need not fear the consumption of a reasonable amount of whole-grain breads and cereals, and can feel free to enjoy the robust health and energy that comes from the sensible eating of such wholesome foods. The regular use of whole-grain products (and/or bran) may have far-reaching health benefits, including prevention of a number of diseases, as well as the potential for alleviating certain diseases already present (as diabetes mellitus and certain bowel diseases).

Foods to Avoid

By now it should be clear from our discussion of the seven major nutritional constituents and the four basic food groups that many excellent foods are available which provide the sound nutrition that is necessary for building and maintaining good health and for preventing disease. It should also be equally clear that we need to avoid many foods which do not provide adequate amounts of the healthful substances which our bodies need.

Candies, pies, cakes, ice cream, and any other "foods" which are loaded with white sugar and white flour, or are otherwise highly refined, should be conscientiously avoided. So should most salty, crunchy, or greasy fried products which are rich in salt, fat, and calories and are generally devoid of nutritional benefit. Sugary carbonated beverages should also be placed on the junk list. Artificially sweetened soft drinks, while not wholesome beverages, may be the lesser among evils for people who are diabetic, obese, or elderly. Any food or beverage that is loaded with preservatives or other chemicals should be avoided as much as possible, especially since some of these chemicals, including saccharin, may prove to have cancer-inducing consequences.

If you are young and healthy, if you exercise regularly and aerobically, and if your diet is basically sound and well-balanced, then a small percentage of junk foods (perhaps 5 percent or less) is probably not particularly harmful. However, elderly or overweight people, or people who suffer from diet-related health impairment, should absolutely avoid all such junk foods. Once junk food becomes part of the daily diet, it becomes nearly impossible to remain within daily caloric limits and still receive adequate nutrients from wholesome foods.

Health Foods

Now we must answer the question, "Is there any value in health foods?" and "Do nutritional supplements improve health?" Most nutritionists feel, at least on a theoretical basis, that no supplements or special health foods are necessary for people who eat a well-balanced diet. However, in real life very few people maintain a truly healthful, well-balanced diet which contains all the necessary nutritional factors in proper balance. For this reason, vitamin and mineral supplements, as well as certain other special food products, may be helpful to many people.

Technically, all nonpoisonous, unprocessed natural foods are "health foods," since they tend to build and maintain health in the normal human body. Fortunately, most such foods that we have been discussing in this chapter are readily available in many supermarkets today. In some areas of the country, whole-grain, whole-wheat bread freshly made without preservatives cannot be purchased from supermarkets, but almost every area of the country has so-called "health food" stores which do carry such products as well as many others (nuts, seeds, vitamin and mineral supplements, etc.)

Special Nutrients

Are organically grown foods highly superior to ordinary supermarket fruits and vegetables? This is a hard question to answer, since present research has not reached clear conclusions on this issue. The organically grown foods may be richer in important trace minerals, and many people are convinced that they definitely taste better. Certainly, foods that have never been fertilized or sprayed with poisons might be considered at least somewhat safer to eat.

Many people would be well-advised to supplement their daily diet with a broad-spectrum vitamin-mineral capsule that contains all the vitamins and minerals (including trace minerals) that are known to be necessary to human health. Vitamin C and B-complex are especially important and might even be taken over and above a multivitamin formula. (But tremendous quantities of Vitamins C and E are not recommended; a good range would be 250 to 1000 milligrams of Vitamin C daily and 200 to 800 international units of Vitamin E daily.) Dolomite powder or tablets provide valuable calcium and magnesium; kelp tablets or powder provide valuable trace minerals; bone meal provides both trace minerals and calcium (but lacks magnesium). Brewer's yeast (*never* baker's yeast) in tablet or powder form provides a valuable spectrum of B-vitamins as well as a number of other important nutrients. (Not all edible yeasts taste the same; try to find one that is at least reasonably palatable.)

Obesity

At the beginning of this chapter we mentioned that the major nutritional problem in the United States and other developed Western nations is the excess consumption of calories with its resulting obesity. This widespread problem is indeed a serious one. Excess weight can lead to a number of health disorders, including high blood pressure, diabetes, gallbladder disease, liver disease, osteoarthritis (degenerative joint disease from excess weight-bearing), some forms of lung disease, and premature coronary heart disease with possible heart attack.

Many Americans are simply eating themselves to death. Frankly, more people are addicted to over-eating than are addicted to alcohol, cigarettes, or drugs. One way to determine if you are overweight is to compare your own weight with the weights listed in the Metropolitan Life Insurance tables for people of light, medium, and heavy frames. Some care is re-quired in determining ideal weights from these tables in so-called light-, medium-, and heavy-framed peo-ple. You may not differ so much in bone structure (perhaps only two pounds or so) but rather in muscle bulk and weight. For example, a very heavily muscled young man with little fat might erroneously be con-sidered overweight by these tables.

Actually, overall appearance and the "skinfold test" may be more reliable than these tables. To use this skinfold test, use your fingertips to probe around your abdomen, buttocks, thighs, and back of the up-per arm to see if you can "pinch an inch." A skinfold thickness greater than one inch indicates excess fat ac-cumulation.

Actuarial studies have shown that, all other things being equal, the people who are least likely to acquire heart disease are those who are actually 10 to 15 percent

DESIRABLE WEIGHTS FOR MEN AND WOMEN
According to Height and Frame, Ages 25 and Over

WEIGHT IN POUNDS (IN INDOOR CLOTHING)

HEIGHT (in Shoes)*	SMALL FRAME	MEDIUM FRAME	LARGE FRAME
MEN			
5' 2"	112-120	118-129	126-141
3"	115-123	121-133	129-144
4"	118-126	124-136	132-148
5"	121-129	127-139	135-152
6"	124-133	130-143	138-156
7"	128-137	134-147	142-161
8"	132-141	138-152	147-166
9"	136-145	142-156	151-170
10"	140-150	146-160	155-174
11"	144-154	150-165	159-179
6' 0"	148-158	154-170	164-184
1"	152-162	158-175	168-189
2"	156-167	162-180	173-194
3"	160-171	167-185	178-199
4"	164-175	172-190	182-204

WOMEN

4 ' 10"	92-98	96-107	104-119
11"	94-101	98-110	106-122
5 ' 0"	96-104	101-113	109-125
1"	99-107	104-116	112-128
2"	102-110	107-119	115-131
3"	105-113	110-122	118-134
4"	108-116	113-126	121-138
5"	111-119	116-130	125-142
6"	114-123	120-135	129-146
7"	118-127	124-139	133-150
8"	122-131	128-143	137-154
9"	126-135	132-147	141-158
10"	130-140	136-151	145-163
11"	134-144	140-155	149-168
6 ' 0"	138-148	144-159	153-173

*1-inch heels for men and 2-inch heels for women.

This table provided by courtesy of the Metropolitan Life Insurance Company, as shown in *Statistical Bulletin*, October 1977. (Derived primarily from data of the *Build and Blood Pressure Study*, 1959, Society of America).

"underweight" by the standards of usual weight tables, such as those provided by the Metropolitan Life Insurance Company.

Losing Weight

In order to be permanently successful in losing weight, a person must first recognize the seriousness of the obesity problem and then resolve to pay the price that is required for permanently losing weight. The person who never admits that he is overweight, and that overweight is a serious problem, and that weight loss requires long-term self-discipline, will never enjoy any appreciable long-term weight loss. Very few overweight problems can legitimately be blamed on metabolic problems, hormonal disorders, or unusual life circumstances; almost all obesity develops from the simple fact of overeating.

Proper, lasting motivation is very important in any weight-loss effort; successful weight loss may require the same kind of fanatical determination needed for giving up smoking, alcohol abuse, or drug addiction. Many people find that their own efforts at weight loss are unsuccessful, and therefore need help from family, friends, physicians, or clinics. Weight Watchers, Diet Workshop, Overeaters Anonymous, and several other weight-loss groups have achieved remarkable success with many of their members.

To the committed Christian there can be a spiritual solution to this problem: prayerfully ask God for help in this matter, recognizing your own failure. Your friends can be of help not only by encouraging you, but also by bearing you up in prayer.

Debatable Tactics

In order to lose weight permanently it is important to go on a reasonable diet and stick to it. Fad diets may help for a few days or weeks, but they are not a long-term solution to the problem of overweight, and such fad diets are sometimes actually dangerous to your health.

For example, diets which consist of only fat and protein do result in weight loss because of hunger depression caused by ketosis or acidosis, but such diets are nutritionally unbalanced and could become dangerous over a period of a few weeks or months. Diets consisting of liquid protein plus water and some vitamin and mineral supplements can indeed produce a remarkable weight loss in a short time, but a number of people using this type of diet have died of serious ventricular arrhythmias (irregular heartbeats), perhaps caused by mineral deficiencies or degeneration of heart muscle induced by this diet. Appetite-suppressing drugs (basically amphetamines) do indeed suppress appetite and result in weight loss, but they tend to be addicting and may also be dangerous for other reasons.

No Easy Road

Let's face it—there is no easy, shortcut road to weight loss. Effective weight loss requires firm personal resolve, a careful, well-balanced diet, and usually aerobic exercise as well.

For dieters who lose weight slowly or not at all, regular vigorous exercise can help remove those pounds that seem reluctant to leave. Brisk walking can result in the burning of 70 to 100 calories per mile. Walking three miles five times weekly could burn 1000 to 1500 calories. This would mean a loss of one pound of fat every two to four weeks, or 15 to 20 pounds a year.

It has been popularly believed that vigorous exercise tends to increase appetite and thereby result in weight gain; however, a number of studies actually appear to show the opposite—that brisk exercise may actually *suppress* appetite, especially in males.

The average active working person could lose weight effectively on a well-balanced diet of 1500 calories daily. Less-active individuals, or active people who want to lose weight more quickly, could use a carefully prepared diet of as few as 1200 or even 1000 calories daily. Below this number, an adequate balance of necessary nutrients becomes almost impossible to maintain. Occasionally an inactive older person will require a reduction to about 800 calories before any significant weight loss takes place, but at this low calorie level proper nutrition is extremely difficult to maintain and can barely be done without special nutritional supplements.

People who are serious about losing weight should certainly eliminate all excess fats, sugars, and empty calories from their diets. For those who feel they must have something sweet, artificial sweeteners like saccharin could be used. (For such people the risk of cancer caused by saccharin intake is far less than the risk of significant obesity with its possible accompanying diabetes.)

Three Meals a Day

Even people on a diet should eat three meals every day, because skipping meals allows for more fat accumulation even when the same daily total of calories is consumed. Also, the regular eating of meals provides a certain sense of sufficiency, helping to prevent compensatory overeating later in the day.

Breakfast could consist of a small-to-medium glass of fruit juice, such as orange juice, or a piece of fruit (perhaps melon), plus a small bowl of cereal containing wheat or bran (with skim milk or low-fat milk). A piece of whole-grain toast could be eaten instead, along with one egg on alternate days, or a glass of skim milk or low-fat milk, and perhaps coffee or tea (but without sugar or cream). There is no place at all for bacon, since it has only one good point (flavor) and four bad features (heavy salt content, heavy fat content, cancer-producing chemicals, and expense—it is one of the most expensive per-pound sources of meat proteins). Processed meats (hot dogs, sausages, cold cuts, etc.), whether eaten at breakfast or any other time, are almost as objectionable as bacon, since such processed products contain much saturated fat, quite a bit of salt, and various kinds of objectionable preservatives, including nitrates and nitrites.

Lunch could consist of a whole-wheat sandwich made up of a small quantity of cheese, tuna fish, unprocessed meat, or perhaps even peanut butter, preferably of the natural variety without added hydrogenated oils. An alternative to the sandwich might include a small bowl of cottage cheese or unsugared yogurt along with a small amount of unsugared fruit or salad. The sandwich lunch could include a glass of skim milk or low-fat milk, but since cottage cheese and yogurt provide some protein as well as calcium and other nutritional factors, this lunch would require no milk drink. If no bread is eaten at lunch, a couple of small whole-grain rye crackers will provide whole-grain nutrition with a minimum of calories. These could be accompanied by a small serving of fruits or vegetables, either cooked or raw, or else low-salt or homemade soup.

For most people the main meal is in the evening, and this is a good time to have a small portion of lean meat, preferably lean ocean fish or else chicken or turkey. This meal could also include potatoes or whole-grain rice along with cooked vegetables and a salad (perhaps with an Italian-type dressing made of corn oil and vinegar.) Dessert is not a requisite of any of these meals.

These examples of three meals could easily total less than 1200 calories daily and still provide well-balanced, nutritious meals which permit effective long-range weight loss. Junky snacks and rich desserts added to any of these meals could of course devastate the caloric advantage of such a careful diet. People who are desperate for between-meal snacks could munch on raw celery or carrot sticks or even a whole-grain rye cracker or two. Wholesome snacks of higher calorie content than these are sometimes appropriate for active growing children or certain adults with diabetes or hypoglycemia.

Fasting

Recently there has been a resurgence of interest in fasting, almost to the point of faddism in some circles. If done under medical supervision and for a restricted period of time, fasting can be an effective means of losing weight quickly. However, prolonged fasting without competent supervision can cause you to lose not only fat but also valuable lean muscle, and can be critically dangerous to your health.

Most people who are overweight but otherwise healthy can handle a fast for one to three days if it is done properly. Occasionally I have personally recommended a modified one-day fast for some of my patients who are on medications for heart disease and high blood pressure and would find it dangerous to fast in the usual way, especially for any prolonged length of time. For such patients I suggest that for one or two days a week (but not on two consecutive days) they eat no regular food but instead take one piece of fruit or one glass of fruit juice three times a day, as well as several glasses of water during the day. This allows for a total calorie intake for that day of about 300 calories or less, yet still provides sufficient fluid and prevents ketosis or acidosis by providing a small amount of natural sugar and sufficient quantities of such critical minerals as potassium. This kind of one-day fast usually entails very little sense of hunger and might be a good way to compensate for a previous bad day of overeating, as happens to many Americans during our major holidays.

All things considered, however, the best way to lose weight permanently is not by fasting, but by sticking conscientiously to a well-balanced, moderate-calorie diet that drops calories safely and permanently.

The Specter of Cancer

Another monstrous problem that may be diet-related is cancer. No word strikes more fear into the hearts of most people than does this word "cancer." If present statistics hold true in the future, one out of four Americans will develop cancer sometime during his or ler lifetime, and one out of five will die of cancer. The cancer problem is indeed an enormous and frightening one.

Federal government studies provide increasing evidence that cancer is caused in large part by pollutants in the air and by chemical substances in our food and drink, and of course by tobacco smoke. A study by the World Health Organization concluded that between 60 and 90 percent of all human cancer is related to environmental factors.

In general, it has been found that people living in heavily industrialized areas, especially near chemical industries, have higher cancer death rates than does the average population. Current estimates indicate that between 15 and 30 percent of all cancer deaths are occupational in origin. Cancers of the lung and chest lining are noted especially among construction and shipyard workers who have been exposed to asbestos. Bladder cancer is noted especially in the aniline dye and rubber industries, cancer of the pancreas especially among organic chemists, and liver cancer especially among workers involved in the manufacture of vinyl and polyvinyl chloride (products used in the plastics industry).

There is increasing general agreement that the American population, especially the work force, has been continuously exposed to both known and unknown chemical carcinogens (cancer-producing agents) in their air, water, and food. For example, carcinogens in many beers, saccharin in many common foods and beverages, and contaminants in many sources of drinking water all contribute to an increased risk of cancer for many Americans.

Self-Influenced Cancer

However, much cancer is self-induced by such bad habits as cigarette smoking. It has been estimated that at least 80 percent of all lung cancer is due to cigarette smoking. Among American males the number one cause of death due to cancer is lung cancer, number two is gastrointestinal cancer (especially colonal rectal cancers), and number three is cancer of the prostate. Among American females the number one cancer killer is now breast cancer, with lung cancer recently moving into second place, and colonal rectal cancer now in third place. Soon lung cancer will probably become the number one killer among females (as among males), since women are now smoking nearly as much as men.

Dietary factors are also important. Excessive consumption of alcohol, and even common obesity, may contribute to cancer. Colonal rectal cancer could be due in large part to a lack of roughage or fiber in the diet, perhaps accompanied by overconsumption of fatty meats, other saturated fats, or even carcinogenic chemicals in commonly consumed foods and beverages, including water. Some researchers feel that supplementary Vitamin C intake every day may help to detoxify some potentially carcinogenic chemicals (such as N-nitroso compounds).

The role of trace minerals, such as selenium and zinc, is under active investigation at this time. Increased intake of certain of such trace minerals, especially selenium, may help to prevent certain kinds of cancers, especially bowel cancer. Trace minerals are theoretically present in adequate quantities in unprocessed natural foods, but since such trace-mineral levels may depend partly on the region of the country in which these foods were grown (because of varying soil richness), trace mineral supplementation may be desirable.

Still Learning

The cause or causes of breast cancer have not yet been clearly identified. Suggested causes include excessive intake of fats and partial deficiencies of certain vitamins or trace minerals. Since a wholesome diet might help prevent breast cancer, and since such a diet is certainly healthful for the whole body, right eating makes sense for everyone. Especially important are balanced proteins and high-quality carbohydrates (in place of refined sugar and processed carbohydrates) as well as decreased fat consumption and increased intake of the trace minerals and Vitamins C, E, and B-complex.

The primary method of preventing most lung cancers is agreed upon unanimously by most researchers—stop smoking! Elimination of carcinogenic dust, smoke, fumes, asbestos, and other air pollutants can also be important as a preventive measure.

Dr. Van Aaken of Germany has hypothesized that vigorous aerobic exercise generally reduces the chance of getting cancer, by increasing the flow of oxygen to all parts of the body. In his survey of middle-aged and elderly people who exercised vigorously, his statistics seem to indicate this kind of correlation.

Although to date not nearly enough is known about effective cancer prevention, we do know that the early detection of cancer is crucial to proper treatment. This is especially true of female cancer of the breast, cervix, and uterus, which can be effectively detected by regular breast examinations, gynecological checkups, Pap smears, and in some cases mammograms.

Even the detection of a bona fide malignancy (true cancer) should not cause total despair, for modern medicine has become increasingly successful in achieving prolonged remissions and sometimes even total cures through modern techniques of surgery, radiation, and chemotherapy.

You Can Do Your Part

As much as 80 percent of all cancer may be preventable by eating properly and avoiding cigarette smoking and environmental pollutants as much as possible. And, of course, right eating carries other rewards: vibrant good health, resistance to cardiovascular diseases, and the enjoyment of a trim figure and clear-thinking mind.

8 THE ULTIMATE JOY

Vibrant physical health is truly a wonderful thing —a highly desirable goal that is realistically achievable for most people. In the previous seven chapters we have seen that, despite the frequent occurrence of such deadly diseases as heart attack, stroke, hypertension, and cancer, our susceptibility to these diseases can be largely overcome by serious dedication to proper diet, vigorous exercise, well-chosen relaxation, and general good-health practices.

But care of the body also pays many dividends for the mind, as even the ancient Greeks recognized in their famous saying, "A sound mind in a sound body." However, there is another crucially important aspect of well-being, beyond the human body and mind, that we have not yet fully considered in this book—the human spirit. Saint Paul's prayer for Christians nearly two thousand years ago was, "May your spirit and soul and body be kept strong and blameless" (1 Thessalonians 5:23, *The Living Bible*). Clearly we are more than animals; our innermost longings can never be fully satisfied by physical health or physical gratification. Nor can mental stimulation alone ever fully satisfy us. Over 1300 years ago Saint Augustine said, ''Thou hast made us for Thyself, O God, and the heart of man is restless until it finds its rest in Thee.''

Today we also may have a restlessness—a void that can only be filled by the God who created us. This important kind of health, with its even higher kind of joy, can be experienced by anyone. You too can have the joy of inner personal peace based on a right relationship with God. While the pursuit of good physical health is a worthy goal, the merit of the pursuit turns into an eternal tragedy if we ignore or reject the personal salvation that is available to us through Jesus Christ.

Much as we may hate to admit it, each of us falls far short of God's perfect standards of inner attitudes and outer behavior, and none of us can adequately atone for past failures by present or future attempts at right living: ''Not by works of righteousness which we have done, but according to His mercy He saved us'' (Titus 3:5); ''For by grace you are saved, by faith, and that not by yourselves; it is the gift of God—not by works, lest anyone should boast'' (Ephesians 2:8,9).

The joy of a right relationship with God begins when we acknowledge our spiritual helplessness in His sight, and then in an act of personal faith acknowledge the crucified and resurrected Lord Jesus Christ as the only answer to the debt of our sins. We are then born again into God's family as His children: "But as many as received Him [Jesus Christ], to them gave He power to become the children of God" (John 1:12). Once we have taken this simple yet profound step, a whole new panorama of enjoyment becomes available to us. We are simultaneously forgiven, justified, redeemed, reconciled, sanctified, and provided with a new kind of faith, hope, love, peace, and joy. And these are just the highlights of a much longer list! We can truly experience the reality of Jesus' words, "I have come that they might have life, and that they might have it more abundantly" (John 10:10), and "Whosoever believeth in Him shall not perish, but have everlasting life" (John 3:16).

Because of the new inner joy and peace which become available to us as part of the salvation package provided by God to all believers, many people who are born again through Christ experience a tremendous alleviation of psychosomatic ailments in their lives. Psychosomatic ailments include bodily pains or other actual physical illnesses induced partly or wholly by mental or emotional attitudes, sometimes unconsciously (subconsciously). Most physicians find that a tremendous percentage of their patients are suffering from ailments that are primarily psychosomatically induced. Guilt, anger, and worry are often major contributors to depression and to various psychosomatic ailments that trouble millions of Americans.

True spiritual conversion is often spectacularly successful in relieving such problems, since a right relationship with God offers tremendous power in dealing with these three tyrants of guilt, anger, and worry, as well as with other problems: "The fruit of the Spirit is love, joy, peace, patience, kindness, goodness, faith, meekness, self-control" (Galatians 5:22,23). True believers—those who are truly born again into God's family—need to recognize that they must continue to depend on God for their spiritual and even their mental and physical well-being. Guilt, worry, anger, depression, and various psychosomatic ailments may afflict a believer who fails to maintain a vital contact with God. We believe that a right relationship with God is vital in obtaining and maintaining vibrant health of spirit, soul (mind), and body.

There is also the great importance, as well as our definite responsibility, of taking care of our physical bodies, as we have outlined in this book. However, there are times when even our best efforts may fail to prevent serious illness. Our God is not only the ultimate Source of all wisdom and knowledge, but He is also the ultimate Source of all healing. The best available medicine and surgery (ultimately God-given) may relieve and even cure our illnesses through the truly astonishing developments of modern medical technology, but even these sources of help can sometimes fail to provide a cure or even very much relief. The believer can be thankful that when illness can be neither prevented nor cured through conventional means, God in His providence sometimes intervenes directly with supernatural healing.

The effect of prayer in a Christian's life is truly powerful, even when God for His own excellent reasons chooses not to bring about healing, either through natural or supernatural means. When good physical health is impossible and suffering becomes inevitable, it is at this time that the born-again Christian has special God-provided comfort, strength, and assurance that is unique to true Christianity. Over the centuries many thousands of true believers have proved the truthfulness of God's promise to believers, "My grace is sufficient for you, for my strength is made perfect in weakness" (2 Corinthians 12:9).

But whether physically healthy, ill, or somewhere in-between, each Christian can rejoice in God's promise of an eternally perfect physical body at the time of the resurrection: [The body] is sown in corruption, it is raised in incorruption; it is sown in weakness, it is raised in power. . . . O death, where is your sting? O grave, where is your victory?" (See 1 Corinthians 15:42,43,55.) Even if a Christian suffers irremedial health problems during this life on earth, he or she will nevertheless revel in perfect physical and spiritual health forever afterwards! Truly salvation through Christ provides the ultimate joy possible in the universe—eternal vibrant health of body, soul, and spirit.